This book is dedicated to Karl Storz, the instrument maker in Tuttlingen West Germany without whose optical telescopes this atlas and countless others would never have been possible.

Clinical Otoscopy
An Introduction To Ear Diseases

Michael Hawke MD FRCS (C)
Professor of Otolaryngology and Pathology,
University of Toronto;
Director, Ear Pathology Research Laboratory;
Otolaryngologist-in-Chief, St Joseph's Health Centre,
Staff Otolaryngologist, Toronto General Hospital, Toronto

Malcolm Keene MB BS (Lond) FRCS
Consultant ENT Surgeon, St Bartholomew's Hospital
and Homerton Hospital, London;
Examiner in Surgery, University of London, UK

Peter W. Alberti MB BS (Dunelm) PhD FRCS (C) FRCS
Professor and Chairman, Department of Otolaryngology,
University of Toronto;
Staff Otolaryngologist,
Toronto General and Mount Sinai Hospitals, Toronto

SECOND EDITION

CHURCHILL LIVINGSTONE
EDINBURGH LONDON MELBOURNE AND NEW YORK 1990

CHURCHILL LIVINGSTONE
Medical Division of Longman Group UK Limited

Distributed in the United States of America by Churchill
Livingstone Inc., 1560 Broadway, New York, N.Y. 10036, and
by associated companies, branches and representatives
throughout the world.

First published 1984
Second edition 1990

ISBN 0-443-04044-3

British Library Cataloguing in Publication Data
Hawke, Michael
    Clinical otoscopy. – 2nd ed.
    1. Man. Ears. Diagnosis. Otoscopy
    I. Title   II. Keene, Malcolm   III. Alberti, Peter W.
    617.8'07545

Library of Congress Cataloging in Publication Data
Hawke, Michael, M.D.
    Clinical otoscopy: an introduction to ear diseases / Michael
Hawke, Malcolm Keene, Peter W. Alberti.—2nd ed.
        p.   cm.
    Bibliography: p.
    Includes index.
    1. Otoscopy.   2. Ear—Diseases—Diagnosis.
    I. Keene, Malcolm.   II. Alberti, Peter W.   III. Title.
    [DNLM: 1. Ear Diseases—diagnosis.   2. Ear Diseases
—diagnosis—atlases.   3. Endoscopy—atlases.
    4. Endoscopy—instrumentation. WV 210 H392c]
    RF123.H39   1990
    617.8—dc20
    DNLM/DLC
    for Library of Congress

Produced by Longman Group (FE) Ltd
Printed in Hong Kong

Preface

The aim of this book is to assist the practitioner in the selection and use of the appropriate equipment when examining the ear, to illustrate the otoscopic appearances of commonly encountered conditions of both the external and middle ear, to outline the aetiology and symptoms of these disorders and to provide the principles and rationale for management.

The accurate diagnosis of any disease depends upon a sound clinical method of examination and the availability of suitable instrumentation to enable a successful examination to be performed. Modern otoscopes which incorporate a halogen light source with fibreoptic distribution of light have greatly improved our ability to illuminate and accurately examine the depths of the external auditory canal.

Today's medical and paramedical curricula place more demands on both students and teachers and consequently there is generally insufficient time and material available to teach an ever increasing number of students the art of clinical otoscopy.

It has become apparent to us, both as teachers and clinicians, that many examiners are unable to appreciate fully the significance of what they see with the otoscope and consequently the diagnosis and management of ear disease is unnecessarily difficult and frequently delayed.

Otoscopy is currently practised by many health care professionals, including audiologists, nurses and nurse practitioners, chiropractors and hearing aid dispensers. With experience and the use of a sound clinical technique, many ear problems can be successfully diagnosed and treated by the primary care provider. We have attempted to emphasize the diagnostic features of those conditions which require specialist referral or surgical intervention.

This colour atlas and text is intended to serve as a practical guide for both physicians and allied health care professionals. We have attempted to provide a fairly complete education in the art of clinical otoscopy and an introduction to otology in general. No attempt has been made to present either a comprehensive atlas of all diseases of the ear nor a complete textbook of otology. By necessity, the text is didactic and the therapeutic advice presented represents our combined clinical experience.

The majority of the illustrations used have been selected from Michael Hawke's personal collection of photographs of the external ear and tympanic membrane. Most of these photographs were taken using a Karl Storz Hopkins rod tele-otoscope with electronic flash and attached endocamera.

In the second edition of this atlas, the text has been expanded and the majority of the colour photographs for the section on diseases of the external ear canal and the section on diseases of the tympanic membrane and middle ear replaced with new slides. A short bibliography has been included for those who wish to refer to more comprehensive texts of otology.

Toronto and London, 1990   MH
MK
PWA

Acknowledgements

We are indebted to many people for their help and advice during the preparation of both editions of this book. The success of any colour atlas depends primarily upon the quality of its photographs. The majority of the photographs in this atlas were taken using a Karl Storz Hopkins rod tele-otoscope which provides the highest quality colour images possible. The Karl Storz photographic system was purchased with a grant from the Richard and Edith Strauss Canada Foundation. Invaluable asistance in the setting up and use of this equipment was provided by Mr Karl Storz, Mrs Sybil Storz-Relling and Mr Hans Joaquim Luneman.

The Ear Pathology Research Laboratory of the University of Toronto has received financial support from many sources over the past years. The financial assistance received from the St Joseph's Health Centre Research Foundation, the TWJ Foundation, Guildford, England, the Saul A. Silverman Family Foundation, The Canadian Otological Study Fund, R. S. Laborie & Associates and Carl Zeiss Jena is gratefully acknowledged. We should also like to express our appreciation to the Ontario Ministry of Health, who supported the Ontario Temporal Bone Bank Programme through a Research Development Grant.

Mr John Senior, Curator of the History of Medicine Museum, Academy of Medicine, Toronto, Audrey B. Davis of the Smithsonian Institute and Miss E. Allen of the Hunterian Museum, Royal College of Surgeons of England provided invaluable assistance in obtaining examples of early otoscopes. Dr Sylvan Stool provided the majority of the historical illustrations for the section on the History of Otoscopy in this edition.

Lou Rednicki and Roger Harris, medical photographers at St Joseph's Health Centre, and Stewart Sereda and Harmiena Van Oosten of the Toronto General Hospital Photographic Department also provided valuable advice and assistance during the preparation of this book.

We would like to thank Lew Allyn and Lorne Elder of Welch Allyn for their enthusiastic support and advice during the preparation of the first edition. Dr Gerald Rosen provided invaluable assistance in the preparation of Chapter 3.

A very special acknowledgement is due to Allison MacKay for her untiring efforts in all aspects of the preparation of this book and especially in the printing of the black and white illustrations. Special thanks are also due to Rasa Skudra, medical artist, for the preparation of the line drawings.

Mr Herb Thony of Carsen of Canada has provided us with valuable technical assistance in the selection and maintenance of our Olympus camera system.

We should also like to record our thanks to our wives and children for their forbearance and encouragement during this project.

Contents

1. The history of otoscopy

You see, gentlemen, that we always come in a dreary circle, again to our starting point, viz. the fact that the profession, up to the present time, have not understood how to examine the ears; such being the case, we must find in this fact, a reasonable ground for the general unsatisfactory condition of the treatment of ear afflictions.
(Anton Von Troltsch 1864 *The diseases of the ear, their diagnosis and treatment*. A textbook of aural surgery translated and edited by D.B. St John Roosa, William Wood & Co., New York.)

INTRODUCTION

Ear disease has afflicted mankind since the days of prehistory. The severe sequelae and deadly nature of certain ear disorders were well known and described in classical Greek, Latin and Arabic medicine, although adequate knowledge of the anatomy of the ear was not forthcoming until more than a millennium later. Appropriate methods of ear examination are of even more recent origin. As with any deep-seated structure, it is necessary to illuminate the area to be examined. The lack of appropriate technology for lighting the depths of the external ear canal delayed the development of instruments for the visual examination of the ear canal and tympanic membrane until the 19th century. The history of otoscopy, the direct inspection of the external canal and tympanic membrane, mirrors the mechanical and technical developments of the 19th and early 20th centuries.

AURAL SPECULA

The first aural specula were devised to help extract foreign bodies from the ear canal, and not to examine the tympanic membrane. Guy de Chauliac, the famous 14th century surgeon, stated in his *Collectorium artis chirurgicalis medicinae*, published in 1363, that 'to diagnose different foreign bodies in the ear canal, it was best to inspect the ear, illuminated by sunlight, with the outer ear canal widened by means of a speculum'. Fabricius Hildanus (1560–1634), city surgeon at Berne (then in Germany), is generally credited with devising the first aural speculum, and modified versions of this same speculum are in use to the present day. He was the first German surgeon to emphasize the need for an accurate knowledge of anatomy. Hildanus also described the neural interconnection between the external ear canal and the larynx which is responsible for the cough reflex occasionally encountered when mechanically cleaning the external ear canal. Hildanus illustrated a bivalve speculum (Fig. 1.1) which was devised to remove foreign bodies from the ear canal. This type of bivalve speculum was in fairly wide use in the 16th and 17th centuries, and came into more general use in the 19th century, being particularly favoured by both Itard and Kramer. By then, specula were being used to examine the tympanic membrane, usually illuminated by allowing sunlight to pass over the examiner's shoulder into the patient's ear. This type of speculum was open to abuse, with some examiners using it in an attempt to over-dilate the ear canal, a most painful and hazardous procedure. The disadvantage of the bivalve speculum is that it requires one hand to keep it open and perhaps the second hand to retract the pinna, thereby preventing adequate

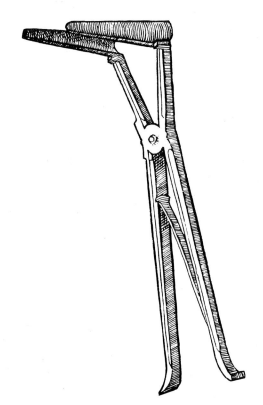

Fig. 1.1 Hildanus's bivalve speculum.

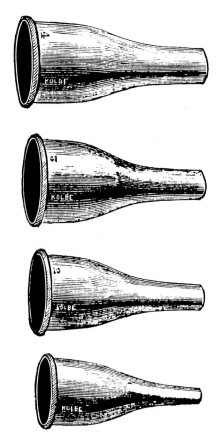

Fig. 1.2 Gruber's aural specula (from Charles H. Burnett 1884 *The ear: Its anatomy, physiology, and diseases. A practical treatise*).

manipulation within the ear. This pattern of speculum is still used today in operative surgery. It is currently known as the Lempert bivalve speculum.

The familiar, simple round or oval specula were not developed until the 19th century. Newberg in 1827 published an article on perforation of the tympanic membrane in which he recommended examining the ear by means of a slender horn tube nearly 10 cm long, with a bell mouth. This instrument was too long to be of practical use but seems to be the origin of the different varieties of tubular specula which subsequently evolved. Dr Ignaz Gruber of Vienna improved upon Newberg's original idea; Gruber's specula are still in use today (Fig. 1.2).

The Irish aurist, Sir William Wilde—who was as famous as his son Oscar—modified Gruber's specula into conical silver tubes $1\frac{1}{2}$ inches (4 cm) long and $\frac{5}{8}$ inches (1.5 cm) wide at their greater aperture and of varying diameter at the medial end which is placed into the external ear canal. Wilde commented that specula should be as light as possible, highly polished both inside and outside, with a stout rim or burr around the larger margin for gripping, and with the smaller (medial) aperture well smoothed so as not to irritate the external ear canal on entering. His specula may also be found in use at the present time.

The English otologist Toynbee was probably the first to make an oval-shaped speculum. Toynbee pointed out that as the normal ear canal was oval in shape it was illogical to insert a round speculum into an oval hole. He also felt that the conical shape of Wilde's specula prevented them

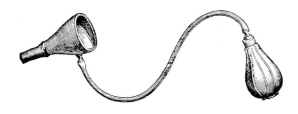

Fig. 1.3 Pneumatic ear speculum of Seigle (from Adam Politzer 1883 *Diseases of the ear*).

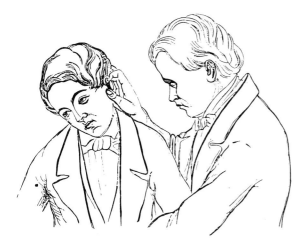

Fig. 1.4 The surgeon examining the external meatus by aid of the sun (from Joseph Toynbee 1860 *The diseases of the ear, their nature, diagnosis and treatment*).

being passed as far as they might be into the ear canal, i.e. they were adequate for the examination of the external portion of the ear but not so good if the examiner desired to see the tympanic membrane.

Politzer, the noted Viennese physician and founder of modern otology, introduced black lucite specula. He felt that this plastic material was warmer, cheaper and the dark colour provided a better contrast with the tympanic membrane than a brightly polished silver speculum. This controversy about the internal colour of specula continues to the present day; the present authors prefer a dark interior.

Siegle (1864) introduced his pneumatic speculum (Fig. 1.3), which consisted of a means of sealing an ordinary aural speculum by glass and a method for alternately applying suction and pressure to the enclosed ear canal and

tympanic membrane. In terms of historical accuracy, this technique had been foreshadowed by Nicolet, a famous Florentine physician, who wrote of one Simeon Seth, who inserted silver or metal tubes tightly into the external canal and sucked upon them in cases of deafness. Simeon was probably a Byzantine physician of the 11th century.

ILLUMINATION

Adequate illumination is of paramount importance in otoscopy. Originally the ear was examined by means of sunlight (Fig. 1.4). Wilde, in the mid 19th century, stated that examinations of the ear should be undertaken, if possible, between the hours of 11 a.m. and 3 p.m. He commented that during the winter months there were many days when there was insufficient light for accurate aural examination. Clearly some form of artificial illumination was necessary.

The first to describe any form of specific illuminator for the ear was Fabricius ab Aquapendente (1537–1619). He described in his *Opera Medica* that in operations on the ear canal it was particularly important to have light falling deeply into the canal. He suggested first that the sun's rays might be allowed to shine through a small hole in the window shade into the ear canal and if this was impossible he used a water-filled flask through which he concentrated the light of a candle.

The English surgeon Cleland, in the 18th century, also recommended a convex glass 3 inches (8 cm) in diameter which could be used to concentrate the beam of a wax candle into the ear canal (Kramer described this as a rude instrument quite inapplicable to practice). This concept was modified by Bozzini, who placed a concave mirror behind the candle.

Little more was achieved until mineral oil lights became available. Both Buchanan, an Englishman, and Kramer devised powerful lights which resembled the magic lantern, consisting of a tin box with a blackened interior provided with a strong lamp, a powerful reflector and convex lenses to concentrate the beam of light. This produced a strong light which, in a darkened room, was thrown into the opening of the meatus.

It is interesting to note that the colour of the ear, when illuminated by artificial light, disturbed the 19th century otologists considerably, for they felt that the normal standard should be daylight and that they could not make accurate observations by artificial light. Over the next 150 years artificial light became the method of choice for the illumination of the ear canal. Now, once again, with the higher colour temperature of modern halogen bulbs, the present generation of otologists is having to learn, in reverse, the lessons of their 19th century forefathers, as this new halogen illumination produces a brilliant light which has a colour temperature approaching that of daylight.

The next major requirement was for an adequate method of directing the light into the depths of the ear canal. Von Troltsch is generally credited with popularizing the use of a mirror in otoscopy, although he himself gives credit to a Dr Hoffman of Westphalia, who in 1841 described the use of a centrally perforated mirror to reflect daylight into the centre of the ear. This concept was not, however, adopted until Von Troltsch came upon the same idea

independently, and showed it in 1855 at the Union of German Physicians at a meeting in Paris. He ultimately fastened the mirror to his forehead (Fig. 1.5) as is currently practised; there were also models of mirrors attached to spectacles, as well as mirrors which were hand-held (Fig. 1.6), models which were an integral part of the artificial light and mirrors which were carefully held in the teeth. The key improvement that this produced was to allow the observer to look down the centre of the beam of light, thereby eliminating head shadow and parallax.

The size and focal length of the mirror was not standardized for some time. Helmholtz had introduced a similar but smaller mirror for the examination of the retina. This was tried by some aurists but deemed too small; others, in an attempt to catch more light, used huge mirrors and only gradually was a diameter of 6–7 cm adopted. The advantage of having a hole in the centre of the mirror is that it provides parallax-free illumination, although even here some of the earlier writers recommended looking alongside the mirror or, for binocular vision,

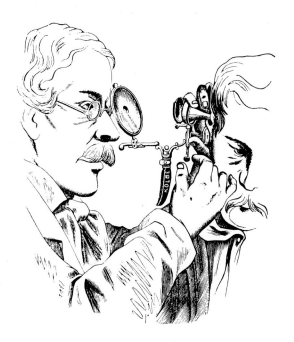

Fig. 1.5 Weber's reflector (from Laurence Turnbull 1887 *A clinical manual of the diseases of the ear*).

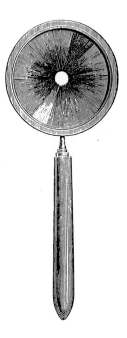

Fig. 1.6 Concave mirror perforated in the centre with handle (from Adam Politzer 1883 *Diseases of the ear*).

described mirrors that were worn in the centre of the forehead with double slots so that both eyes could be used—a system that can still be found today in certain electric headlights. The focal length of the mirror for otoscopy was originally 5–6 inches (13–15 cm), much shorter than is presently used. It was only after otology and laryngology became united that a universal mirror with a focal length of about 12–13 inches (30–33 cm) was adopted for use in both laryngoscopy and otoscopy.

The use of a mirror to collect and focus light gave a new lease to daylight as a means of illuminating the ear canal and by the 1880s the accepted way of examining the ear was by means of daylight (Fig. 1.7), preferably from a northern aspect, concentrated by means of a head mirror and shone directly into the ear canal.

Otologists used a wide variety of lighting devices for the examination of the ear well into the early part of the 20th century. These included a mineral oil lamp, even the lowly candle (Fig. 1.8), gas mantles and, best of all, limelight because of its brightness and similar colouring to daylight. However the latter source was difficult to use, and found only in clinics. Gradually electric light was introduced, both in the form of fairly powerful bulbs, the light of which could be concentrated by lenses on to a head mirror, such as the McKenzie bull's-eye lamp which is still in use today, and in the form of smaller, low voltage bulbs which could be placed directly into an otoscope or on to a headband. The miniature bulb was not perfected until the early part of the 20th century.

The principle of the dry cell battery was known in the 1860s; however a reliable product was not commonly available until the First World War and was not applied in any routine way to the manufacture of portable otoscopes until the efforts for the war were concluded. Thus, it was not until the early 1920s that reliable small bulbs and dependable easily obtainable flashlight batteries made the otoscope, as we know it today, a practical proposition.

THE OTOSCOPE

By the late 19th century the stage was set for the combination of mirror and speculum into one instrument. The idea of using a perforated mirror set in a cylinder at an angle of 45° to the cylinder with an ear speculum at its end came to several aurists simultaneously, including Bonnafont and Brunton who had instruments manufactured in their name. With these teaching

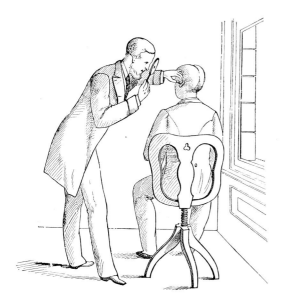

Fig. 1.7 Method of examining the auditory canal and tympanic membrane (from St John Roosa 1881 *A practical treatise on the diseases of the ear*). Photograph courtesy of Dr S. Stool.

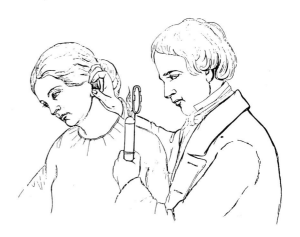

Fig. 1.8 The surgeon examining the external meatus by means of Miller's lamp and the tubular speculum (from Toynbee 1860 *The diseases of the ear*).

otoscopes the observer looked directly into the ear canal along the straight axis and through the perforated mirror while the patient and observer sat at right angles to a window or source of artificial light which was caught by the mirror and reflected into the ear canal. This was the basis of Bonnafont's (Fig. 1.9), Brunton's (Fig. 1.10), and Toynbee's illuminating (Fig. 1.11) otoscopes. The latter was the more commonly used and remained in the catalogues until well into the 20th century.

Brunton's auriscope was first described in an article which appeared in the *Lancet* in 1865. This auriscope worked on the principle of a periscope: light from a candle or lamp was concentrated by a funnel and then reflected by a plane mirror set at an angle of 45° into the ear canal. The mirror had a central perforation through which the examiner could view the ear.

Brunton's otoscope could be, and was, fitted with a magnifying lens for the observer and could also be sealed with plain glass at the illuminating end. It was thus possible to alter the pressure within by means of a small rubber tube into which the observer sucked or blew while observing the movement of the tympanic membrane, thereby emulating Siegle's pneumatic otoscope.

Brunton's otoscope was much in use amongst general practitioners but was decried by otologists because it denied them a means of manipulating in the ear canal—a dichotomy which continues to the present day with family practitioners being avid users of the otoscope and specialists using head mirrors and specula or operating microscopes when manipulation within the ear canal is necessary.

There was adequate room in a Brunton otoscope for a light bulb and consequently these

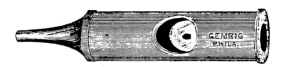

Fig. 1.9 Bonnafont's otoscope (from Charles H. Burnett 1884 *A treatise on the ear*).

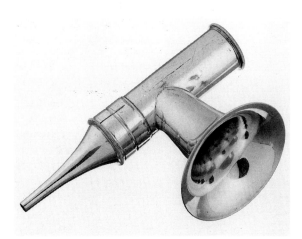

Fig. 1.10 Brunton's auriscope c. 1880 manufactured by J. Wood, Spurriergate, York, England.

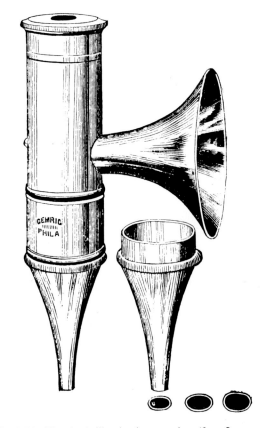

Fig. 1.11 Toynbee's illuminating speculum (from L. Turnbull 1887 *A clinical manual of the diseases of the ear*). Photograph courtesy of Dr S. Stool.

were the first otoscopes to be electrically illuminated. There was a German model produced by Schall in the 1890s and a Spanish model invented by Verdos of Barcelona in 1895. In any event, this device was further modified from its original dependence upon wet cells to flashlight batteries and was in continuous production as a portable auriscope until the early 1930s. It again became available in a modified form in the late 1960s as the Hotchkiss otoscope. James Hinton, the eminent Victorian aurist, added a teaching observer attachment to Brunton's otoscope (Fig. 1.12). This is mirrored in a recently introduced teaching head for a modern American (Welch Allyn) portable otoscope (see Fig. 2.9, p.13).

Otoscopes have been produced with small magnifying lenses so that instruments can be introduced through the speculum into the ear canal, with large magnifying lenses that pneumatically seal the speculum so that a Siegle attachment can be used, and with specula of various shapes and materials, both reusable and disposable, imitating the designs of their 19th century predecessors in metal and plastic.

Recent developments have included improvements in illumination by means of miniature halogen bulbs which produce a brighter, whiter light, and the introduction of fibreoptic illumination, which brings an even circle of light close to the tip of the otoscope. This, too, is but a modern improvement of Blake's operating otoscope of nearly 80 years ago which used a prism in a similar way. Modern specula have sponge rubber seals which allow an airtight fit for pneumatic otoscopy.

MICROSCOPY

No history of otoscopy would be complete without some comment on the use of the ear microscope. In 1872, Dr de Rossi of the University of Rome claimed to have invented a binocular otoscope which resembled in many ways the Helmholtz ophthalmoscope—in a sense, a binocular loop with a very long working distance. As ear surgery became more precise with the development of the fenestration operation and then stapedectomy, a binocular operating microscope became essential. And although various instruments were adapted, none came into routine use until after the Second World War. The widespread use of the Zeiss operating microscope, available since approximately 1950, has revolutionized ear surgery and has now had many modifications and many imitations. It is mentioned because, although introduced for operating room use, its value in the clinic quickly became evident. Such operating microscopes are now in routine use for outpatient otoscopy in most major centres and many private offices throughout the world.

THE TELE-OTOSCOPE

In 1966, Karl Storz realized the optical potential of making telescopes using a unique rod lens system that had been invented by the English physicist Professor H. Hopkins. This system utilized a series of long cylinders of optical quality glass which have lens surfaces on each end. These rod lenses are positioned in such a way that spaces which act as air lenses are created between the ends of the rods. The result of this Hopkin's rod air lens system is a higher degree of brightness, resolution (sharpness) and greater depth of field than could be obtained with conventional telescopes. In addition the optical diameter of the rod lens system can be made very small to enable extremely thin instruments to be manufactured while maintaining high optical

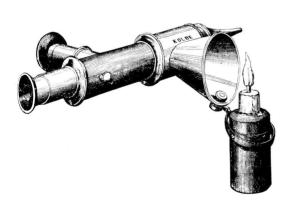

Fig. 1.12 Hinton's modification of Toynbee's illuminating speculum which allows both physician and student to see at the same time (from Turnbull 1887 *A clinical manual of the diseases of the ear*). Photograph courtesy of Dr S. Stool.

quality. This is obtained by the large aperture of the rod lens system which enhances image brightness.

The Hopkin's rod tele-otoscope created and manufactured by Karl Storz has completely revolutionized photography of the external ear canal, tympanic membrane and middle ear. Most of the colour photographs in this book were taken with a 4 mm diameter Karl Storz Hopkins rod tele-otoscope.

2. The instruments

BASIC PRINCIPLES

The tympanic membrane is situated deeply within the head, at the medial end of the only skin-lined canal in the body, the ear canal. In order to examine the tympanic membrane it is necessary to illuminate adequately the entire recess. This difficulty can be largely overcome if a sufficiently brilliant form of illumination is used and if the tortuous external auditory canal is straightened out to bring the tympanic membrane into view.

In the past, illumination has been traditionally provided by electric light reflected into the ear by a perforated head mirror. This method provides coaxial illumination, which allows the examiner to look along the path of the beam of light, while freeing both of the examiner's hands to hold the aural speculum and instruments. The tortuosity of the mobile outer cartilaginous external ear canal is straightened and the deeper bony canal and tympanic membrane are exposed by means of an aural speculum inserted into the outer external auditory canal.

The addition of magnification allows a more accurate inspection and assessment of the ear to be carried out. The binocular operating microscope currently represents the state of the art, since it incorporates both variable magnification and stereoscopic (three-dimensional) vision while freeing both of the examiner's hands for instrumentation and manipulation within the ear canal. Unfortunately, the operating microscope is a large and relatively expensive instrument; its use is generally restricted to the specialist in the clinic, consulting room or operating theatre.

Over the past century, a succession of portable otoscopes (auriscopes) incorporating battery powered electric bulbs have been introduced and the electric otoscope is nowadays by far the most commonly used instrument for examination of the ear. These small and portable otoscopes are easy to use and convenient, although manipulation of the ear through the otoscope head is somewhat limited and technically more difficult.

THE HEAD MIRROR (Fig. 2.1)

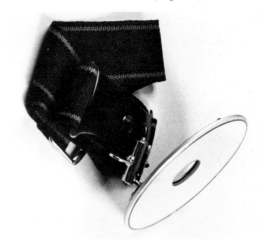

Fig. 2.1 Perforated head mirror with webbing forehead band (Downs Bros, Church Path, Mitcham, Surrey CR4 3VE, UK).

The majority of head mirrors are $3\frac{1}{2}$ inches (89 mm) in diameter, with a central aperture approximately $\frac{3}{4}$ inch (19 mm) in diameter. The concavity of the mirror is designed to concentrate the source of light at a distance or focal length of $7\frac{1}{2}$ inches (190 mm). Various models of head mirrors incorporating adjustable headbands of webbing, fibre or polyethylene are available.

The goose-neck joint between the mirror and the headband is an essential feature which enables the mirror to be easily adjusted. The mirror should be large enough to concentrate light, but not so large that it obstructs vision by the other eye. The primary advantage of the head mirror is that it is light and portable, and, if well designed, the illumination provided is very bright.

Its successful use does, however, depend on the availability of a suitable bright light source. Although a naked 100 W electric bulb is sufficient for most purposes, a special lamp fitted with a halogen bulb and a condensing lens is preferred by many examiners because of the increased brightness of this newer type of light source.

THE ELECTRIC HEADLIGHT (Fig. 2.2)

An electric headlight, worn on the centre of the forehead just above the bridge of the nose, is preferred by many physicians. The electric headlight is easier to position accurately because the beam of light moves in unison with the examiner's head. Most headlights are adjustable and should be capable of producing an evenly illuminated circle of light. In the modern headlight, this is achieved by adjusting an iris diaphragm. For the majority of applications a light spot of $1\frac{1}{2}$ inches (37 mm) is optimal. Many modern headlights incorporate a quartz halogen lamp which produces significantly brighter illumination with no filament shadows. One slight disadvantage of most headlights is the absence of coaxial illumination. This problem has been overcome by some manufacturers by the incorporation of a perforated mirror for illumination; through this mirror the examiner may view the area being observed.

Both the head mirror and the headlight enable the examiner to inspect the ear stereoscopically while leaving both hands free for instrumentation and manipulation.

AURAL SPECULA (Fig. 2.3)

A suitable speculum is required to hold open the outermost portion of the cartilaginous meatus and to allow the passage of both light and instruments. As a general principle, the largest aural speculum which can be comfortably

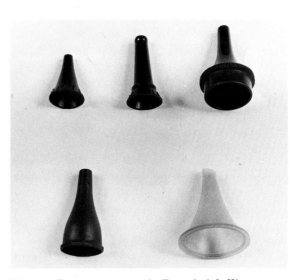

Fig. 2.3 **Top**: otoscope specula. From the left: Kleenspec, a disposable speculum for use with a fibreoptic otoscope; a polypropylene reusable speculum for use with a fibreoptic otoscope; a polypropylene speculum for use with the older diagnostic or operating otoscope. **Bottom**: traditional specula. Left: a metal speculum; right: a polypropylene Shea type of operating speculum.

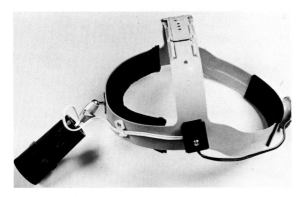

Fig. 2.2 Electric headlight powered by a wall transformer (Welch Allyn, Inc., 4341 State Street Road, Box 220, Skaneateles Falls, NY 13153-0220, USA).

introduced into the meatus should be used. The appropriate size for adults is from 4 to 7 mm in diameter; for children it is approximately 3 mm and for infants a speculum as small as 2 mm may have to be used. Because the normal external canal is oval rather than circular in cross-section, oval specula tend to fit more easily and snugly into the canal than those which are perfectly round.

With the patient seated, an oval speculum is inserted with its widest diameter in the vertical axis. The ideal speculum is smooth and has a non-reflecting dark inner surface. Specula made either of metal (expensive) or synthetic plastic materials (inexpensive) are available. There are many inexpensive plastic specula which, for safety and convenience, can be discarded after a single use. This type of speculum can, however, be reused after careful washing to remove all visible debris, and sterilization by autoclaving or by immersion in a suitable cold antiseptic solution. One excellent example of this type of plastic speculum is the Shea type of operating speculum available from Richards Surgical (Memphis, Tennessee).

THE ELECTRIC OTOSCOPE (AURISCOPE) (Fig. 2.4)

An electric otoscope must be capable of delivering light of sufficient brilliance to illuminate fully the depths of the external ear canal. Until recently, the standard source of illumination has been an incandescent bulb mounted axially to allow sufficient light to emanate from the end of the speculum. This design has two inherent drawbacks: the position of the bulb interferes with instrumentation through the otoscope, and the smallest departure from its optimal position greatly reduces the amount of light emerging from the end of the speculum. If the instrument is inadvertently dropped or mishandled, the bulb carrier can easily become misaligned and it is hardly surprising that some students of otoscopy experience difficulties when handed an instrument which is incapable of adequately illuminating the ear canal.

To avoid this obvious pitfall, examiners are encouraged to obtain and look after their own instruments and 'neither a borrower nor a lender be'!

When purchasing this type of classic otoscope, care should be taken to ensure that the bulb and bulb carrier are correctly centred and that the maximum possible light is being delivered through the speculum.

Those modern otoscopes (Fig. 2.4) which incorporate a halogen light source and fibreoptic circumferential light distribution are generally superior. Halogen illumination produces a very bright light with a higher colour temperature, which allows a more accurate observation of subtle changes in tissue colour. The light intensity of the modern quartz halogen bulb is three times that of an ordinary incandescent bulb, and the light output remains consistently high over the entire life of the bulb.

The examiner should always be aware that the perceived colour of the ear canal and tympanic

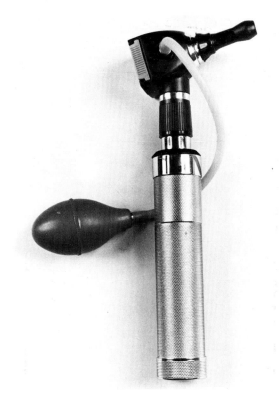

Fig. 2.4 3.5 V halogen fibreoptic pneumatic otoscope and throat illuminator (Welch Allyn 20 000) with rechargeable battery handle (Welch Allyn 71 000).

membrane will vary according to the type of light source used. A new series of norms must be learned if changing from incandescent to halogen light or vice versa. The colours observed when using an otoscope equipped with a halogen light resemble those seen when the ear is illuminated with a head mirror reflecting sunshine or bright northern daylight (see Chapter 1).

The fibreoptic transmission or distribution of light provides a 360° ring of light without visual obstruction or reflections from the interior of the speculum. Those otoscopes which are illuminated by an incandescent bulb utilize a 2.5 V power supply. Those modern otoscopes which are illuminated by the brighter quartz halogen light bulbs require a 3.5 V power supply.

The otoscope head can be powered by disposable dry batteries, rechargeable nickel cadmium cells (Fig. 2.5) or from an a.c. (mains) transformer. The voltage required is determined solely by the characteristics of the bulb fitted to the instrument. The power source for the otoscope should incorporate a variable rheostat to enable the examiner to adjust to optimum the brilliance and colour temperature of the light.

Whereas the voltage available from ordinary dry cells decreases consistently with use, a

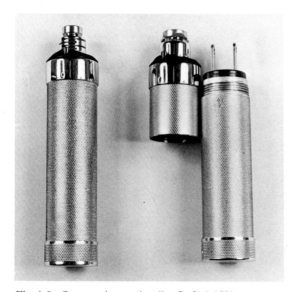

Fig. 2.5 Otoscope battery handles: **Left**: 2.5 V battery handle for C size cells (Welch Allyn 70 500). **Right**: a wall rechargeable 3.5 V handle (Welch Allyn 71 000).

rechargeable nickel cadmium battery handle eliminates frequent battery changes and provides a relatively uniform voltage output almost to the end of discharge. The most convenient of rechargeable handles plug directly into an a.c. (mains) outlet and will recharge automatically if left overnight.

OTOSCOPE HEADS

Otoscope heads can be broadly divided into those with which pneumatic otoscopy is possible (closed systems) and those which are unsuitable for pneumatic otoscopy (open systems).

Four patterns of otoscope heads are commonly available:

1. Standard diagnostic pneumatic otoscope.
2. Fibreoptic pneumatic otoscope.
3. Operating otoscope.
4. Teaching head.

Standard diagnostic pneumatic otoscope (Fig. 2.6)

This traditional older model features an enclosure so that when the speculum is introduced into the ear canal a closed air chamber is created between the external canal and the interior of the otoscope (closed system). The standard diagnostic otoscope features coaxial illumination which can be derived either from an incandescent bulb (2.5 V system) or a halogen light source (3.5 V system). By attaching a valveless rubber bulb to a side arm or opening in the enclosure, pneumatic otoscopy is possible. The excellent illumination combined with the wide bore of the speculum makes the Welch Allyn 3.5 V halogen standard diagnostic otoscope (Fig. 2.6; Welch Allyn 20 200) the otoscope of choice for both the routine examination of the ear and pneumatic otoscopy.

Fibreoptic pneumatic otoscope (Fig. 2.7)

The most modern otoscope head designs feature a fibreoptic light distribution. This is accomplished by incorporating a ring of light-conducting fibres within the shell of the otoscope; these fibres provide a 360° ring of light, thereby eliminating visual obstruction by the light bulb as well as reducing internal reflections.

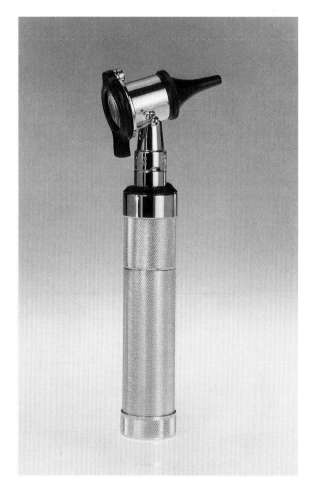

Fig. 2.6 3.5 V halogen diagnostic pneumatic otoscope head (Welch Allyn 20 200). This is the preferred otoscope for both routine examination and pneumatic otoscopy.

Specially designed specula slip over the nose of the instrument. By sliding the wide-viewing lens to one side, instruments can be introduced through these otoscopes.

Operating otoscope (Fig. 2.8)

The operating otoscope which incorporates a small rotatable magnifying lens was designed to facilitate access and instrumentation into the external auditory canal. The speculum holder can be adjusted in relationship to the fixed coaxial light source. Pneumatic otoscopy is not possible with this open type of system.

Teaching head (Fig. 2.9)

Based on Brunton's original design of 1862, the teaching otoscope incorporates two magnifying viewing ports which allow simultaneous observation of the ear by the examiner and an observer. This design is useful for instruction and demonstration to students and patients' relatives.

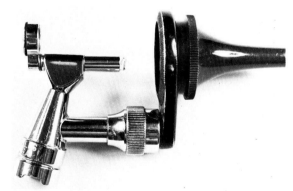

Fig. 2.8 2.5 V operating otoscope head (Welch Allyn 21 600).

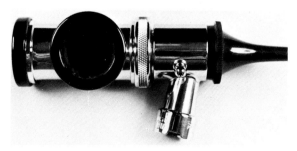

Fig. 2.9 3.5 V halogen teaching otoscope head (Welch Allyn 20 202).

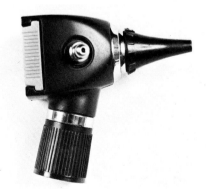

Fig. 2.7 3.5 V halogen fibreoptic pneumatic otoscope and throat illuminator (Welch Allyn 20 000).

PRESBYOPIA AND THE OTOSCOPIST

Otoscopic examination cannot be performed successfully unless the examiner's eyes can focus sharply on the structures examined with the otoscope. With advancing age (usually starting around the fourth decade), the eyes lose their ability to accommodate and become farsighted due to a combination of ciliary muscle weakness and a loss of elasticity in the crystalline lens of the eye. The presbyopic otoscopist may find some difficulty in bringing the tympanic membrane sharply into focus when viewing through the otoscope.

This problem can usually be resolved by varying the length of the speculum used or by wearing corrective eyeglasses. It is hoped that in the future, some farsighted manufacturer will provide corrective lenses (ranging in power from +3 to −3 dioptres) that can either be clipped on to the back of the otoscope or inserted in place of the standard magnifying lens (the standard lens varies from +9 to +11 dioptres) provided with the otoscope.

OTOSCOPE SPECULA (Figs 2.3 and 2.10)

Most otoscopes incorporate specula which are conical in shape and have round openings. The authors strongly recommend polypropylene reusable specula which are well shaped and practical to use. Specula with parallel sides are generally to be avoided, because they unnecessarily limit the field of view. With an appropriately sized hand-held speculum, the tympanic membrane can be clearly seen. Whenever magnification is used, the field of view is diminished and the examiner must learn to move the otoscope systematically around to observe all of the tympanic membrane and develop a composite view.

When pneumatic otoscopy is to be performed, the use of a Sofspec speculum (Welch Allyn) is helpful (Fig. 2.10). These specula have soft flanged tips which fit snugly into the ear canal and provide a superior seal for pneumatic otoscopy.

In addition, the soft flange provides increased comfort to the patient and a significant degree of protection against damage to the external canal.

THE TELE-OTOSCOPE (Fig. 2.11)

The tele-otoscope is a miniature telescope modelled on the cystoscope; it enables the specialist to inspect and photograph the tympanic membrane. Modern versions of these instruments use the Hopkins rod lens system which incorporates glass rods separated by air-filled gaps, acting as lenses, placed at specific intervals along the teleotoscope. Tele-otoscopes provide the observer with a wide viewing angle, excellent resolution, contrast and brilliant illumination. The larger angle of view provides a circumferential image of the entire tympanic membrane through a teleotoscope with an overall diameter of only 2.7 mm. Tele-otoscopes are

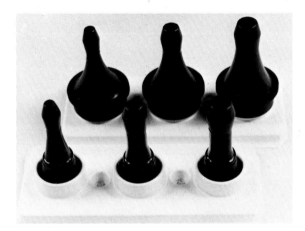

Fig. 2.10   Sofspec specula for standard diagnostic heads (Welch Allyn 22 120; **top**) and fibreoptic heads (Welch Allyn 24 420; **bottom**) †.

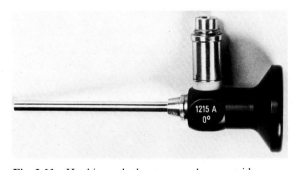

Fig. 2.11   Hopkins rod tele-otoscope: 4 mm outside diameter (Karl Storz model 1215A; Karl Storz GmbH & Co., Mittelstrasse 8, D-7200 Tuttlingen, West Germany).

unfortunately costly, and consequently are not in general use.

THE OPERATING MICROSCOPE (Fig. 2.12)

The binocular operating microscope, although primarily designed for microsurgery of the ear, is also a valuable diagnostic tool. The operating microscope fulfils all the requirements necessary for adequate otoscopic examinations. With excellent illumination and stereoscopic optics, the examiner enjoys increased depth perception and three-dimensional vision, and is thus able accurately to manipulate instruments introduced through a speculum. The majority of operating microscopes permit changes in magnification to be made either by a rotating drum or by a zoom lens system.

The attachment of a beam splitter to the microscope body allows the addition of supplementary optics. These may include observer eye pieces, a still camera body, a cine camera or even a colour television camera, thereby simplifying the teaching and documentation of ear disorders. For consulting room use, simple wall-mounted versions of the operating microscope are now available.

THE AUDIOSCOPE (Fig. 2.13)

The audioscope (Welch Allyn) is an otoscope which has fibreoptic illumination, and which incorporates a screening audiometer. The audiometer produces pure tones at 500, 1000, 2000 and 4000 Hz with an intensity of 25 dB.

For audiometric screening, special tips (audio tip; Welch Allyn) must be used in order to ensure that the intensity of the tone generated is accurate.

For better visualization of the tympanic membrane the examiner may wish to use a speculum with a larger central bore.

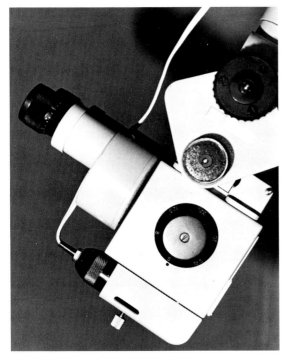

Fig. 2.12 Zeiss-Jena operating microscope model OPMI 2. (Veb Carl Zeiss Jena, 1 Carl Zeiss Strasse, Jena, GDR).

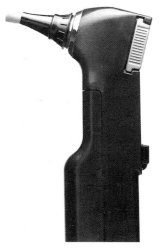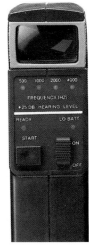

Fig. 2.13 The audioscope (Welch Allyn).

THE MICROTYMP (Fig. 2.14)

Tympanometry provides an objective measurement of middle ear function by measuring sound reflected from the tympanic membrane while the pressure in the external ear canal is changed from a positive pressure of 200 dPa through normal atmospheric pressure to a negative pressure of −300 dPa.

The MicroTymp is a small, hand-held portable automatic tympanometer (impedance audiometer) which is shaped like an otoscope, and which provides an objective measurement of middle ear function in 3 seconds and displays the results on a liquid crystal display. The graphic display from each ear can be stored in memory and when the test is completed a permanent hard copy of the test can be printed out for the records.

ADDITIONAL INSTRUMENTS

A small number of additional instruments are necessary to deal with conditions commonly encountered during the examination of the ear.

Aural syringe (Fig. 2.15)

A metal aural syringe of the Wood or Simpson pattern is recommended for general use. Both conical metal pipes and the Toynbee pipe with a smooth bulbous tip are quite satisfactory. A relatively inexpensive polypropylene ear syringe is now available which has a smooth action and is leak-free. A Bacon pattern aural syringe is lighter in use and has the advantage of being self-charging (self-filling). Many European otologists prefer a rubber Higginson syringe fitted with a soft rubber nozzle. A suitably shaped receiver or ear trough is required to catch the effluent.

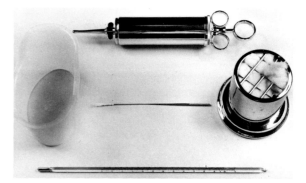

Fig. 2.15   Instruments required for syringing.

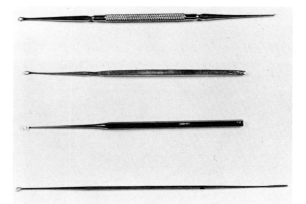

Fig. 2.16   Curettes and probes. **From above:** Formby cerumen scoop; Hovell fine silver loop; Buck blunt ear curette and Jobson Horne probe.

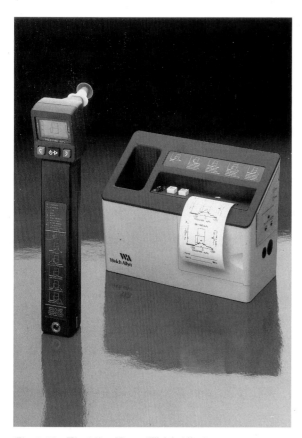

Fig. 2.14   The MicroTymp (Welch Allyn).

Curettes and probes (Fig. 2.16)

A selection of blunt wax hooks, curettes and probes are necessary for the removal of wax and foreign bodies from the ear canal. We have found the Jobson Horne probe, the Buck blunt ear curette and the St Bartholomew's Hospital blunt hook to be particularly useful. In inexperienced hands, a sharp wax hook or curette can easily traumatize the delicate canal skin. The Jobson Horne probe doubles as a cotton wool carrier or, alternatively, a silver Hunter–Todd probe may also be used as a cotton-tipped applicator.

Aural suction (Fig. 2.17)

Soft wax, smooth foreign bodies, purulent debris and water are best aspirated from the ear canal using an angled aural suction tip of either the Bellucci or Zoellner pattern. Number 3 and number 5 French gauge are the most suitable sizes.

Culture kit (Fig. 2.17)

Sterile pre-packed kits (Fig. 2.17) are convenient for culture studies of material removed from the ear canal. Most of these incorporate a suitable transport medium, such as Stuart's transport medium, so that even if the swab is delayed on the way to the laboratory an accurate specimen of pathogenic bacteria or fungal micro-organisms will still be obtained.

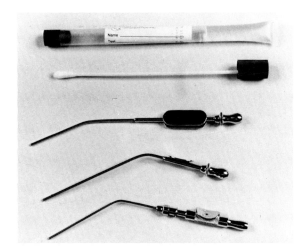

Fig. 2.17 Culture kit and suction tubes. **From above:** two-part culture kit; Zoellner suction tube; Bellucci suction tube; Verhoeven suction tube with House cut-out adapter.

Aural forceps (Fig. 2.18)

Wilde's aural forceps with serrated points are satisfactory for the majority of applications. A pair of Hartmann crocodile-action forceps with serrated jaws are extremely useful for removing extruded tympanostomy tubes (grommets) from the external auditory canal. In addition, a pair of cup forceps are useful for biopsy purposes.

GENERAL ENT INSTRUMENTS (Fig. 2.19)

When a complete examination of the ear is necessary, attention must also be paid to the upper air and food passages. A Lack tongue depressor, a suitable nasal speculum, a selection

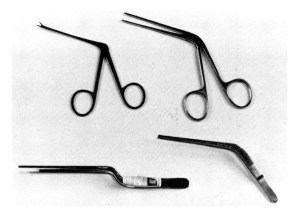

Fig. 2.18 Grasping forceps. **Clockwise from top left:** Hartmann's crocodile action forceps; Tilley aural forceps; Wilde aural forceps; bayonet-shaped nasal dressing forceps.

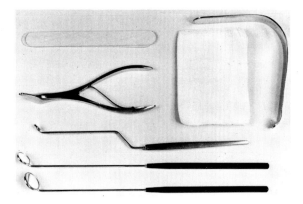

Fig. 2.19 General ENT examination instruments. Lack tongue depressor, Pilcher nasal speculum, St Clair Thomson nasopharyngeal mirror and two laryngeal mirrors.

of nasopharyngeal and laryngeal mirrors, together with a means of preventing these mirrors from misting, such as a spirit lamp or suitable anti-fog solution, should be available. Some examiners favour a warming device which contains electrically heated glass beads.

To undertake simple clinical tests of hearing and balance (Fig. 2.20) a 512 and a 1024 Hz tuning fork, a Bárány noise box for masking the opposite ear, a Dundas Grant tube and a 1 ml tuberculin syringe for instilling iced water into the external canal will be required.

A rubber stamp with a schematic diagram of the right and left tympanic membrane is extremely useful for recording clinical observations (Fig. 2.21).

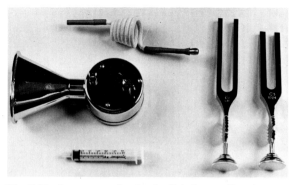

Fig. 2.20   Instruments for simple clinical tests of hearing and balance. **Clockwise from top left**: Dundas Grant coil; Gardiner Brown tuning forks (512 and 1024 Hz); 1 ml disposable syringe for caloric stimulation; Bárány noise instrument with cone.

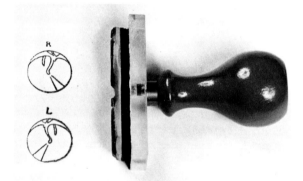

Fig. 2.21   Tympana documentation stamp.

3. Clinical anatomy of the ear

An understanding of the basic anatomy of the ear is necessary both for the appreciation of the normal appearances of the ear and the understanding of those disorders of structure and function which result from disease processes.

For anatomical purposes, the ear can be conveniently divided into three parts—the *external* ear, the *middle* ear and the *inner* ear.

Only the external ear and the tympanic membrane are normally accessible for direct examination, unless the tympanic membrane is perforated or absent, in which case a number of the important middle ear structures may be seen. The inner ear, which is situated deeply within the temporal bone (Fig. 3.1), houses the end organs of hearing and balance (Fig. 3.2) and cannot be inspected directly.

THE EXTERNAL EAR

The external ear consists of the *auricle* (which includes the pinna and the lobule), the *external auditory canal* (meatus) and the outermost layer of the *tympanic membrane* (drum-head).

The auricle is a convoluted leaf of irregularly shaped elastic cartilage which is covered by skin and attached to the lateral aspect of the head. The elastic cartilage which supports the pinna (except at the lobule) is continuous with the cartilage of the outer portion of the external auditory canal. The important anatomical

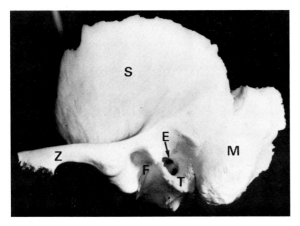

Fig. 3.1 Lateral view of the left temporal bone. The squamous portion (S), the mastoid portion (M), and the tympanic ring (T) are visible. The bony external auditory canal (E), is situated just behind the glenoid fossa (F) of the temporomandibular joint. The zygomatic process (Z) projects anteriorly.

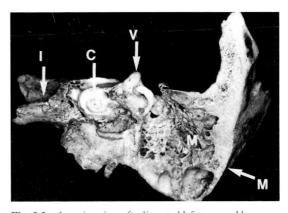

Fig. 3.2 Anterior view of a dissected left temporal bone. The bony otic capsule located within the petrous pyramid is displayed. The dense white bone of the cochlear (C) and vestibular (V) parts of the otic capsule stand out quite clearly. The entrance of the internal auditory canal (I) and the mastoid process (M) filled with air spaces are also shown. Photograph courtesy of Dr Chung-Ling Peng.

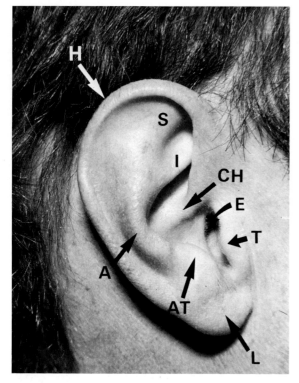

Fig. 3.3 Anatomical landmarks of the external (right) ear. The helix (H), the lobule (L), the tragus (T), the antitragus (AT), the antihelix (A), the superior (S) and inferior (I) crura of the antihelix, the crus of the helix (CH), and the external auditory meatus (E) are shown.

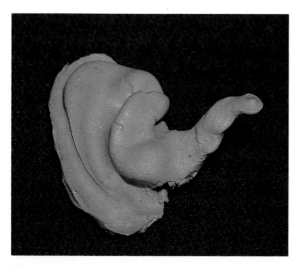

Fig. 3.4 The tortuous shape of the external auditory canal and the oblique angle at which the tympanic membrane is set in respect to the central axis of the canal can be seen in this cast of the pinna and entire external canal.

features of the auricle are illustrated in Figure 3.3.

THE EXTERNAL AUDITORY CANAL

The external auditory canal—the only blind-ending, skin-lined canal in the body—is 24 mm long in the adult and barely wide enough to admit a pencil. The lumen of the canal is ovoid in cross-section with the long axis of the oval lying in the vertical plane. The external auditory canal follows a tortuous course (Fig. 3.4) from the conchal bowl inwards to reach the tympanic membrane.

The superficial or outer third of the canal (cartilaginous external auditory canal) is surrounded by cartilage and runs backwards and upwards.

The deep or inner two-thirds of the external auditory canal (bony external auditory canal) has bony walls (Fig. 3.5) and initially runs slightly backwards before turning to run forwards and downwards. The narrowest portion of the canal (*the isthmus*) is found at the junction between the outer cartilaginous third and the bony inner two-thirds.

The skin lining the outer cartilaginous canal (Fig. 3.6) is relatively thick, containing hairs and both sebaceous and modified apocrine (ceruminous) glands. The underlying cartilaginous framework allows the outer cartilaginous canal a moderate amount of mobility.

In contrast, the skin overlying the inner bony two-thirds of the external canal is thin and contains neither hair nor glandular structures (Fig. 3.7). It is closely adherent to the underlying bone (Fig. 3.8) and consequently the skin which lines this area is both immobile and easily traumatized.

It is important to note that the skin covering the outer aspect of the tympanic membrane is continuous medially with that lining the deep canal and laterally with the more complex outer skin of the external ear.

The epithelium covering the surface of the tympanic membrane and external auditory canal possesses a unique self-cleansing mechanism. The outer, most superficial layers of corneocytes of the skin in this area desquamate by migrating radially off the surface of the tympanic membrane and then laterally along the bony canal to the outer cartilaginous canal where the superficial keratin is shed into the ceruminous material. This mechanism accounts for the normal self-cleansing action of the ear and can be observed by following, over a period of weeks, the path of the scab produced by a myringotomy incision. One of the risks of using a cotton bud to clean the ear is that it just pushes wax and debris back into the ear.

The external ear is innervated by branches of several cranial nerves; the trigeminal (V), the facial (VII), the glossopharyngeal (IX) and the vagus (X), together with branches of the second

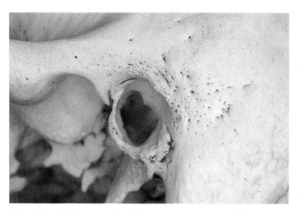

Fig. 3.5 The bony walls of the deep external auditory canal can be seen in this dried temporal bone specimen. The tympanic bone makes up the greater part of the bony canal.

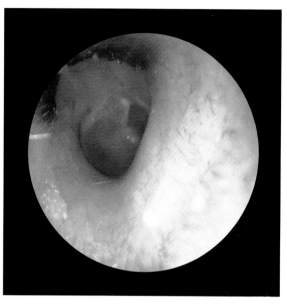

Fig. 3.7 The bony external auditory canal (right ear). Notice the thinness of the skin and absence of hairs within the bony external auditory canal. The posterior bulge of the anterior canal wall partially obscures the anterior portion of the tympanic membrane.

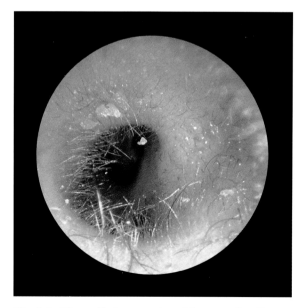

Fig. 3.6 The cartilaginous portion of the external auditory canal (right ear). Notice the numerous tiny villus hairs within the cartilaginous portion of the external auditory canal. Large terminal hairs are often encountered in adult males.

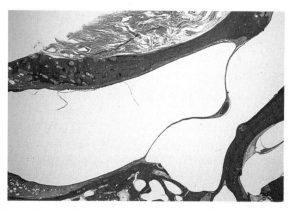

Fig. 3.8 This horizontal temporal bone section shows a portion of the thick skin of the superficial canal, the entire bony canal and the tympanic membrane.

and third cervical sensory roots. With this diverse nerve supply, it is not surprising that many conditions affecting the upper food and air passages can present as pain referred to the ear.

TYMPANIC MEMBRANE (DRUM-HEAD)

The tympanic membrane is a pale grey, ovoid, semi-transparent membrane, positioned obliquely at the medial end of the external auditory canal. In section it is conical, like a loud-speaker. The tympanic membrane is formed of three layers—an outer epithelial layer which is continuous with the skin of the bony external auditory canal, a fibrous supporting middle layer, which gives the tympanic membrane its strength and shape and an inner mucosal layer, which is continuous with the mucosal lining of the tympanic cavity.

The lower four-fifths of the tympanic membrane contain a well organized fibrous middle layer called the pars tensa. In the upper fifth of the tympanic membrane the pars flaccida (Shrapnell's membrane) has a sparser, less organized middle layer and is consequently more mobile.

The fibrous middle layer of the pars tensa, which contains two layers of fibres— circumferential and radial fibres—is attached to the handle of the malleus, which can be seen extending downwards and backwards, ending at the apex of the triangular cone of reflected light (Fig. 3.9). The long process of the incus and its articulation with the head of the stapes may frequently be seen through the posterosuperior quadrant of a thin normal tympanic membrane.

The chorda tympani nerve which supplies taste to the anterior two-thirds of the tongue is sometimes visible in the posterosuperior quadrant, passing horizontally across the middle ear just behind the tympanic membrane between the long process of the incus and the handle of the malleus (Fig. 3.9).

The anterior portion of the tympanic membrane derives its nerve supply from the auriculotemporal branch of the trigeminal nerve; the posterior portion of the tympanic membrane and the floor of the external canal are innervated by the auricular branch of the vagus nerve (Arnold's nerve). The medial surface of the

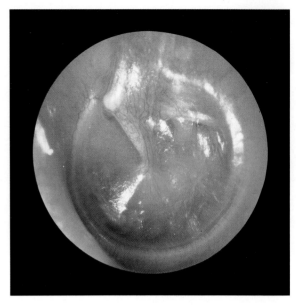

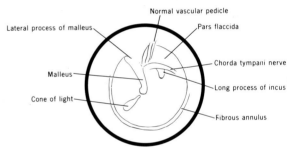

Fig. 3.9 Normal thin tympanic membrane (left ear). Notice the detail of the normal blood vessels running along the handle of the malleus. The end of the long process of the incus is just visible in the posterosuperior quadrant.

tympanic membrane is innervated by the tympanic branch of the glossopharyngeal nerve (Jacobson's nerve).

The lateral aspect of the tympanic membrane derives its blood supply from both the circumferential and the manubrial branches of the deep auricular branch of the maxillary artery (Fig. 3.10). In the normal state, the tympanic membrane appears almost avascular, but after a prolonged examination of the ear, syringing, crying, or in inflammatory conditions, these vessels may become quite prominent.

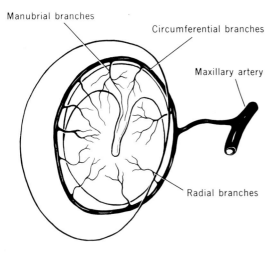

Manubrial branches

Circumferential branches

Maxillary artery

Radial branches

Fig. 3.10 Blood supply of the tympanic membrane (right ear). The tympanic membrane receives a major portion of its blood supply from the maxillary artery via the deep auricular branch. There is a ring of circumferential blood vessels just lateral to the annulus. Numerous radial branches pass from this circumferential ring across the tympanic membrane.

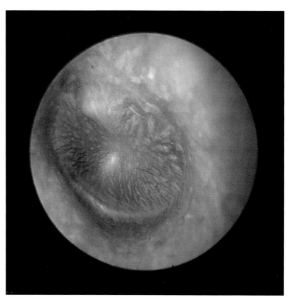

Fig. 3.11 Note the white patches of thickened keratin scattered over the pars tensa of this normal tympanic membrane.

Keratin patches (Fig. 3.11)

If the tympanic membrane is examined with sufficient illumination, multiple discrete thickened whitish patches can be seen. These patches consist of tiny stacks of keratinocytes which have developed as the superficial layers of keratin split apart during their normal outward migration. Keratin patches are present on the surface of all normal tympanic membranes, although they may not always be visible. Maceration of the outer surface of the tympanic membrane by moisture or oedema of the tympanic membrane, for example during an acute otitis media, usually enhances their visibility.

The shape and distribution of keratin patches can be clearly demonstrated by staining the surface of a cadaveric tympanic membrane with 1% osmium tetroxide (Fig. 3.12). The osmium stain is taken up by the keratin patches, staining them black.

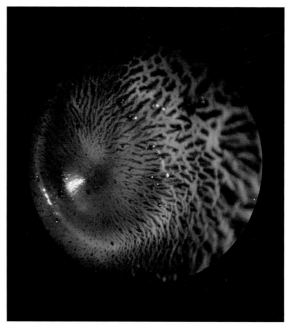

Fig. 3.12 The keratin patches on the pars tensa of this cadaveric specimen appear black after staining with osmium.

Transverse wrinkles of the deep canal (Fig. 3.13)
Another normal feature of migration which is frequently encountered is a series of transverse wrinkles in the superficial layer of corneocytes of the deep bony external auditory canal. These transverse wrinkles are surface corrugations or waves which lie at right angles to the long axis of the external canal. Transverse wrinkles are present in most deep canals and they are most readily visible on the posterior surface. These wrinkles develop as the outwardly migrating stratum corneum of the deep canal is heaped up against the stationary adnexal structures, especially the hairs, of the superficial canal. Transverse wrinkles become larger and more numerous as the migrating epithelium of the deep canal approaches the junction between the deep and superficial portions of the external canal (the deep–superficial junction).

THE MIDDLE EAR CLEFT

The middle ear cleft consists of a series of interconnected air-filled cavities which are located within the temporal bone. The middle ear cleft comprises the eustachian tube, through which the middle ear cleft obtains its air supply; the tympanic cavity (middle ear); the mastoid antrum, which connects the tympanic cavity to the mastoid air cells, and the mastoid air cell system.

The tympanic cavity is approximately 15 mm in height and length. It resembles a flattened box set on edge, with a pipe emerging from its narrow front wall—the eustachian tube (Fig. 3.14).

The anterior wall contains openings for the entry of two structures—the tensor tympani muscle and the eustachian (pharyngotympanic) tube. The eustachian tube runs anteriorly and medially from the tympanic cavity to the nasopharynx and is responsible for the normal aeration of the middle ear cleft.

A large potential defect in the outer surface of the box is covered by a mobile membrane—the tympanic membrane. The area inside the box which lies above the level of the tympanic membrane is the attic or epitympanum; that below the membrane is the hypotympanum and that directly medial to the tympanic membrane is the mesotympanum.

The floor of the middle ear is a thin layer of bone which separates the tympanic cavity from the carotid artery and the jugular bulb. The roof of the tympanic cavity, the tegmen tympani, separates the tympanic cavity from the contents of the middle cranial fossa (the meninges and overlying temporal lobe of the brain).

The posterior wall of the box features a depression which contains the short process of

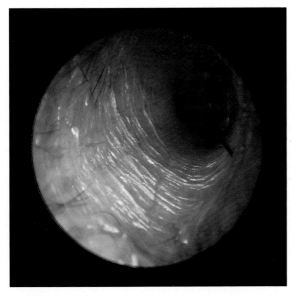

Fig. 3.13 Note the heaped-up wave-like transverse wrinkles on the floor of this normal bony external auditory canal.

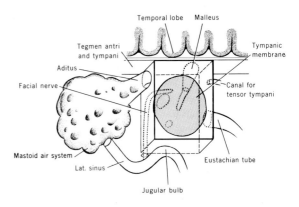

Fig. 3.14 Schematic box diagram showing the structures adjacent to the middle ear cavity (right ear).

the incus (the fossa incudis) and admits the chorda tympani nerve into the middle ear space. Posterosuperiorly the mastoid antrum connects the tympanic cavity to the mastoid air cell system. The stapedius muscle arises from a small pyramidal eminence situated at the junction of the posterior and medial walls.

The medial wall of the middle ear is also the lateral aspect of the inner ear. The most prominent landmark is an outward bulge—the promontory—which covers the basal turn of the cochlea and encroaches into the middle ear space to within 2 mm of the tympanic membrane.

There are two apertures in the medial wall of the middle ear which communicate with the inner ear—the oval window which is occupied by the stapes footplate, and the round window which is covered by a thin membrane (the round window membrane).

The tympanic ossicles

The three tympanic ossicles—the malleus, the incus and the stapes—the smallest bones in the body, span the middle ear and connect the tympanic membrane to the oval window of the bony labyrinth of the inner ear (Figs 3.15 and 3.16). Together, these three ossicles are referred to as the ossicular chain.

The malleus (hammer), the outermost ossicle, is 9 mm in length and consists of three parts—a rounded head situated in the attic and hidden from otoscopic view, a neck, and a handle embedded in the upper half of the tympanic membrane which has a short process protruding from its lateral aspect.

The middle ossicle, the incus (anvil), is tooth-like in appearance and consists of a body and two diverging processes. The body of the incus lies in the attic, where it articulates with the head of the malleus. The short process extends backwards into the fossa incudis and is attached to it by a ligament. The long process, which may be seen through the posterosuperior quadrant of a thin tympanic membrane, descends

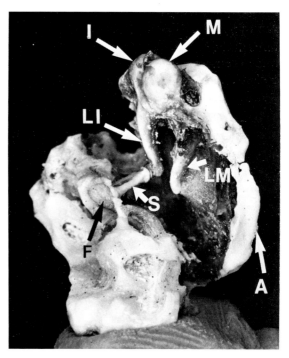

Fig. 3.16 A dissection of the ossicular chain. The head of the malleus (M) and the body of the incus (I) are located in the epitympanum. The long process of the incus (LI) is seen articulating with the head of the stapes (S). The stapes footplate (F) is visible in the oval window niche.

The long process (handle) of the malleus (LM) is attached to the tympanic membrane. A small part of the bony annulus (A) has been left to support the tympanic membrane. Photograph courtesy of Dr C.L. Peng.

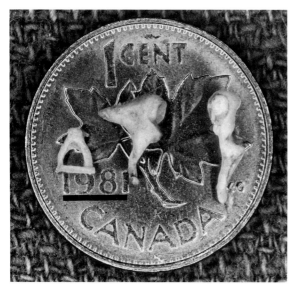

Fig. 3.15 The ossicles. The stapes, incus and malleus are displayed from left to right upon a Canadian 1 cent coin. The black line underneath the date is 5 mm in length.

medially and terminates in a knob, the lentiform process, which articulates with the head of the stapes.

The smallest and most medially placed ossicle, the stapes (stirrup) is composed of a head, neck, diverging crura or limbs and a footplate. The head articulates with the incus and the footplate sits in the oval window niche of the bony inner ear.

The tympanic muscles

Two tiny muscles—the tensor tympani and the stapedius—insert into the ossicular chain. The tensor tympani, which is innervated by a branch of the mandibular division of the trigeminal nerve (V), is inserted into the upper end of the malleus handle. Contraction of the tensor tympani muscle pulls the malleus and tympanic membrane medially.

The body of the stapedius muscle, which is innervated by a branch of the facial nerve (VII), is completely enclosed within the bony pyramid, with its tendon emerging to be inserted into the posterior aspect of the head of the stapes. The stapedius tendon can occasionally be seen through a posterior perforation of the tympanic membrane. Contraction of the stapedius muscle tilts the stapes footplate in the oval window, decreasing its mobility.

The tympanic plexus

This plexus of nerves is derived chiefly from the tympanic branch of the glossopharyngeal nerve (IX) and from branches of the sympathetic plexus of the internal carotid artery. It lies beneath the mucous membrane on the promontory of the medial wall of the tympanic cavity, where it can occasionally be seen through a defect in the tympanic membrane. The tympanic plexus sends branches to the mucous membrane lining the middle ear cleft and gives off secretomotor fibres that eventually reach the parotid gland.

THE INNER EAR

The inner ear is located deeply within the petrous part of the temporal bone and is beyond the range of the otoscope. However, modern diagnostic imaging techniques have improved our ability to inspect this region, thereby enhancing our understanding of the effects of both congenital and acquired disorders of hearing and balance. A knowledge of the basic anatomy of the inner ear is required to appreciate both the mechanisms of normal inner ear function and the paths by which structural changes can result from diseases arising in the middle ear cleft or surrounding regions.

The inner ear consists of two parts—the bony labyrinth (Fig. 3.17) and the membranous

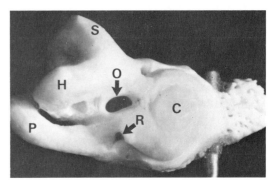

Fig. 3.17   The bony otic capsule of a right ear has been dissected. The cochlea (C) is located anteriorly. All three semi-circular canals—superior (S), horizontal (H) and posterior (P)—can be clearly seen. The oval window (O) from which the stapes footplate has been removed and the round window niche (R) are also clearly visible.

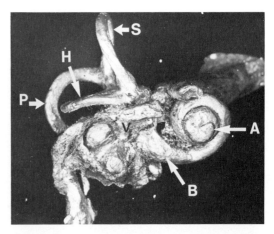

Fig. 3.18   A lead cast of the interior of the bony labyrinth. The apical turn of the cochlea (A) and the basal turn (B) are clearly visible. The vestibule (V) lies just posterior to the cochlea. The superior (S), horizontal (H) and posterior (P) semi-circular canals are also defined. Photograph courtesy of Dr C. L. Peng.

labyrinth (Fig. 3.18), which lies within but does not completely fill the bony labyrinth.

The bony labyrinth

The bony labyrinth is composed of the vestibule, the three semi-circular canals and the cochlea. The vestibule, which is situated between the middle ear and the internal auditory canal, communicates with the semi-circular canals posteriorly and the cochlea anteriorly. The vestibule communicates with the middle ear by means of two windows in its lateral wall—the oval window which is occupied by the stapes footplate, and the round window which is covered by the thin round window membrane.

Each of the three semi-circular canals (superior, lateral and posterior) forms two-thirds of a circle and has a small swelling (the ampulla) at one end.

The cochlea resembles a snail shell, enclosing a central canal 30 mm long which spirals for $2\frac{3}{4}$ turns around a central pillar, the modiolus (Fig. 3.19). The basal turn of the cochlea forms the promontory of the medial wall of the middle ear. The osseous spiral lamina winds around the modiolus like a screw thread and separates the cochlear canal into the scala vestibuli (running from the oval window) and the scala tympani (running to the round window). These two compartments are filled with perilymph and communicate with each other through the helicotrema, a small hole in the osseous spiral lamina near the apex of the cochlea.

The membranous labyrinth

The membranous labyrinth (Fig. 3.20), which is

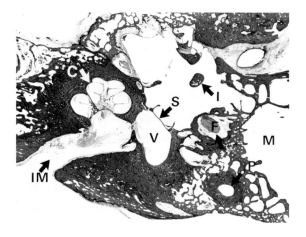

Fig. 3.19 A mid modiolar horizontal section of a (right) human temporal bone. The internal auditory meatus (IM) is seen leading toward the cochlea (C) and the vestibule (V). The stapes footplate (S) is seen filling the oval window. A portion of the long process of the incus (I) is visible within the middle ear. The facial nerve (F) and the posterior semi-circular canal (P) are also visible. There are numerous air cells within the mastoid process (M).

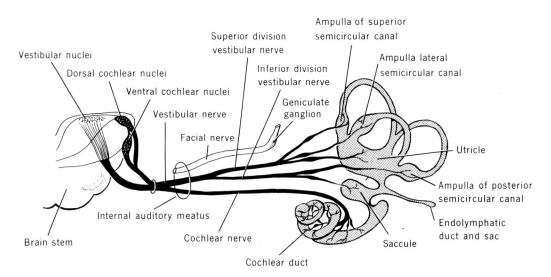

Fig. 3.20 Schematic diagram of the membranous labyrinth and its innervation.

filled with endolymph, consists of the utricle, the saccule, the three semi-circular ducts and the cochlear duct. The space between the membranous and bony labyrinths is filled with perilymph.

Each of the three membranous semi-circular ducts—the horizontal (lateral), the superior (vertical) and the posterior—contains a bulbous swelling (the ampulla). A tiny sense organ, the crista (Fig. 3.21) is situated within each ampulla.

The utricle receives the five openings of the semi-circular ducts and communicates with the saccule. Both the saccule and the utricle also contain sense organs (maculae; Fig. 3.22).

The cristae and the maculae contain modified sensory neuroepithelium which is innervated by branches of the vestibular nerve. Ducts from the utricle and the saccule join to form the endolymphatic duct which terminates under the dura on the posterior surface of the petrous temporal bone as a dilatation—the endolymphatic sac. The ductus reuniens connects the lower part of the saccule to the cochlear duct, which then spirals upwards, ending blindly at the apex. The cochlear duct (scala media) divides the cochlea into the scala vestibuli and the scala tympani. The basilar

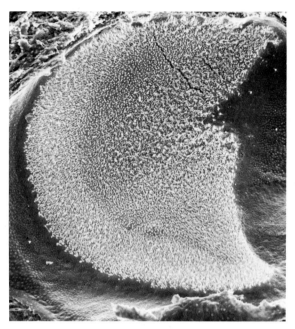

Fig. 3.22   The macula of the utricle. SEM view of the macula of the utricle of a chinchilla. The statoconial layer has been removed so that the striola can be seen as an area of less dense sensory cells with shorter stereocilia. Photograph courtesy of Dr I. Hunter-Duvar.

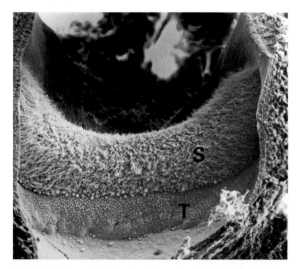

Fig. 3.21   A vestibular crista. Scanning electron microscope (SEM) view of the side of the crista of a chinchilla. Notice the saddle shape of the crista. The transitional cell area (T) can be seen next to the sensory cells (S). Photograph courtesy of Dr I. Hunter-Duvar.

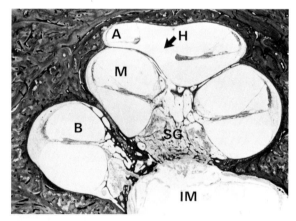

Fig. 3.23   A mid modiolar section of a human cochlea. The three turns of the cochlea—the apical (A), the middle (M), and the basal (B)—can be seen. The helicotrema (H), through which the scala vestibuli and scala tympani communicate, is seen in the apical turn. The spiral ganglion cells (SG) are located within the middle of the cochlea or modiolus. The internal auditory meatus (IM) is located at the base of the cochlea.

membrane extends from the osseous spiral lamina to the outer wall of the bony labyrinth. Reissner's membrane runs obliquely from the osseous spiral lamina to the lateral wall of the bony labyrinth, dividing the cochlear duct from the scala vestibuli (Figs 3.23 and 3.24).

The organ of Corti (the spiral organ of hearing) consists of a group of modified neuroepithelial cells overlying the basilar membrane (Fig. 3.25). The pillar cells form a tunnel which divides the organ of Corti into inner and outer parts. A single row of hair cells is present on the inner side and three rows of hair cells are present on the outer side. The hair cells project stereocilia into the overlying tectorial membrane. Nerve fibres in contact with hair cells pass through the spiral lamina to the spiral ganglion within the modiolus and thence to the internal auditory canal as the cochlear nerve. The auditory pathway then continues via the brain stem to reach the higher auditory centres of the cerebral cortex.

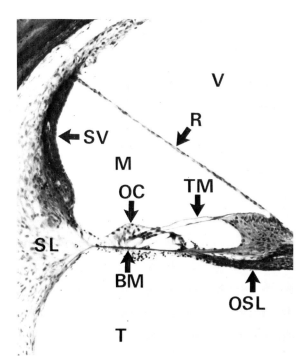

Fig. 3.24 A high-powered photomicrograph of a human temporal bone section. Details of the middle turn of the cochlea are demonstrated. The three compartments of the cochlea, the scala vestibuli (V), the scala media (M) and the scala tympani (T), can be seen. The scala vestibuli is separated from the scala media by Reissner's membrane (R). The stria vascularis (SV) is located on the outer wall of the scala media. The organ of Corti (OC) is situated upon the basilar membrane (BM). The tectorial membrane (TM) lies upon the top of the outer hair cells of the organ of Corti. The basilar membrane and the osseous spiral lamina (OSL) divide the scala media from the scala tympani. The spiral ligament (SL) is seen lateral to the organ of Corti.

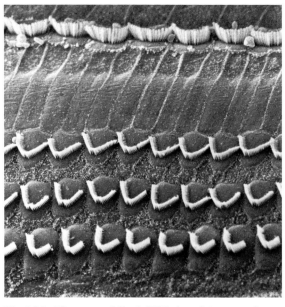

Fig. 3.25 The organ of Corti. SEM view of the top surface of the human organ of Corti. The stereocilia of the single row of inner hair cells and the three rows of outer hair cells are clearly shown. Photograph courtesy of Dr I. Hunter-Duvar.

4. Physiology of the ear

The ear is a specialized sense organ with two basic functions. These are the perception of sound (hearing) and the detection of changes in posture and spatial orientation (balance). Both senses rely on adaptation of primitive vibration detectors, and share many similarities.

PHYSIOLOGY OF HEARING

For descriptive purposes the auditory portion of the ear can conveniently be divided into two parts (Fig. 4.1)—a *sound-conducting apparatus* consisting of the external ear, the tympanic membrane, the ossicular chain and the

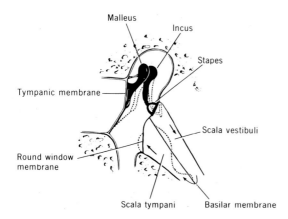

Fig. 4.1 Diagrammatic view of the sound-conducting mechanism. *Note*: As sound energy displaces the stapes footplate *inwards*, the wave of pressure passing through the scala vestibuli to the scala tympani causes the round window membrane to bulge *outwards* and induces vibration of the basilar membrane.

labyrinthine fluids (which conduct the airborne sound vibrations to the inner ear with a minimal loss of energy), and an *electromechanical transducer* which transforms mechanical sound energy (vibrations) into nerve impulses which are then transmitted to the auditory cortex of the brain, where they are perceived as hearing. This can be likened to a microphone, which converts (transduces) mechanical vibration into an electrical impulse. The ear is like a biological microphone; like a microphone it takes sound vibrations and converts them into an electrical signal—a nervous impulse. However it is a biological microphone, deep in the head, bathed in body fluids. It has therefore developed a complex mechanism to conduct sound from the surrounding air through the outer and middle ear to the inner ear with minimal energy loss.

Sound travels as a wave consisting of an alternating compression and rarefaction of the molecules in the medium through which it is propagated or travels, e.g. air or water. In the region of compression the pressure of the air is slightly higher than normal, whereas in the region of rarefaction the pressure is slightly lower than normal. When the source of the sound stops vibrating, the propagation of these pressure variations stops, and the medium returns to its normal pressure.

Sound waves may be physically quantified in terms of frequency and amplitude. The brain's subjective perception of these parameters is referred to as pitch and loudness respectively. The exact mechanism by which the inner ear and its central connections perform this function is not completely understood, and is outside the scope of this book.

The sound-conducting apparatus

The sound-conducting apparatus consists of the external ear, the tympanic membrane, the ossicular chain and the labyrinthine fluids. The external ear consists of the pinna (auricle), external auditory canal and the epithelial layer of the tympanic membrane.

Although the pinna is not as prominent in man as in many other animals, it nevertheless has several important functions. The shell-like shape of the conchal bowl serves to collect, amplify and funnel sound down the external auditory canal. It has an important function in localizing the origin of sounds.

The external auditory canal conveys sound to the tympanic membrane and affords a considerable degree of protection to the tympanic membrane and the delicate contents of the middle ear.

The middle ear sound-conducting mechanism consists of the tympanic membrane and ossicular chain, which absorb airborne sound waves and transmit them with little loss of energy to the relatively dense fluids of the inner ear. Since air and water present greatly differing resistance to the passage of sound energy (impedance), the middle ear conducting mechanism has evolved as a transformer, thereby overcoming this impedance mismatch. The pressure of sound waves arriving at the tympanic membrane is increased 18-fold at the stapes footplate. This is achieved by a combination of an areal difference and a lever effect.

The acoustic energy collected by the relatively large area of the pinna is in turn transmitted down the ear canal to the tympanic membrane. Here it is absorbed and transmitted to the smaller area of the stapes footplate (the hydraulic effect). In addition, the ossicular chain acts as a lever with a mechanical advantage of 1.3 to 1. The net effect of these two mechanisms (14×1.3) is a gain of approximately 18 to 1. The amplitude of vibration at the stapes footplate is reduced compared to that of the tympanic membrane, while the force per unit area transmitted to the labyrinthine fluids is increased by a similar ratio.

The intratympanic muscles

The stapedius muscle provides a degree of protection to the delicate hair cells of the cochlea, by contracting in response to loud sound. By limiting the excursion of the stapes footplate at the oval window, the amount of acoustic energy reaching the inner ear fluids is reduced. In normal individuals this contraction occurs reflexly at sound pressure levels of 80–90 dB above threshold.

The tensor tympani muscle dampens vibration of the ossicular chain, thereby preventing an uncomfortable acoustic reverberation.

The eustachian tube

The pressure changes produced by sound waves are so small that the tympanic membrane must be free to vibrate efficiently. In order to do so, the air pressure on both sides of the membrane must be the same; think of the reduction of hearing produced by an unequal pressure differential when you have a cold. The eustachian tube provides the mechanism which equalizes the air pressure in the middle ear to that of the surrounding atmosphere.

The eustachian tube is the only route by which air can enter or exit the normal middle ear. The eustachian tube is responsible both for the maintainance of normal middle ear ventilation and for pressure regulation. The air within the tympanic cavity is constantly and slowly absorbed by the mucosa lining the middle ear cleft. The middle ear transformer mechanism is only able to operate at peak efficiency if the air pressure is identical on both sides of the tympanic membrane. If this absorbed air is not replaced, over time a negative pressure will develop in the middle ear and the tympanic membrane will be pulled inwards (retracted). If this negative intratympanic pressure persists, eventually the middle ear cleft will become filled with a serous fluid.

The eustachian tube is normally closed to prevent the sound of normal nasal respiration and that of one's own voice from passing up the eustachian tube and into the middle ear. The eustachian tube normally opens only on swallowing or yawning. These brief but repetitive periods of eustachian tube opening are sufficient to maintain normal middle ear aeration. A failure of normal eustachian tube function is responsible for a significant proportion of acquired middle ear disorders.

The inner ear sound-conducting mechanism

The inner ear portion of the sound-conducting mechanism transmits acoustic energy from the stapes footplate, situated in the oval window, to the perilymph of the scala vestibuli. This acoustic pressure wave then passes up the scala vestibuli, deforming the membranous labyrinth. The round window membrane moves in an opposite phase to the stapes footplate, thus allowing the incompressible perilymph to move in the rigid bony labyrinth: as the stapes footplate rocks inwards, the round window membrane bulges outwards into the middle ear cavity. As the sound pressure wave travels through the perilymph along the cochlear duct, a secondary vibration of the basilar membrane is produced (Fig. 4.1).

The sensorineural transducer

Pressure waves passing through the perilymph induce a travelling wave in the basilar membrane. The peak of the wave (the area of maximum displacement) varies with the frequency of the sound: the higher the frequency of the sound, the closer to the stapes footplate lies the peak of the travelling wave. These movements of the basilar membrane set up a shearing action upon the hair cells, whose stereocilia are embedded in the tectorial membrane. This deformity leads to an excitation of the afferent nerve fibres; a nervous impulse is propogated and relayed along the auditory pathway to the auditory cortex of the brain. The hair cells which respond to high-frequency sounds are situated in the basal turn of the cochlea, whilst those responding to lower frequencies are located in the middle and apical turns. While there are several current theories, the precise mechanism by which the cochlea encodes both the frequency and intensity of sound into neural impulses is not yet clearly understood.

The vestibular labyrinth

The maintenance of body posture and equilibrium (balance) depends upon the integration of sensory input from three main systems—the eyes, the proprioceptive system of the muscles and joints and the vestibular apparatus of the inner ear. The vestibular system may be divided into two parts—a peripheral component formed of the vestibular end organs with their nerves, and a central component consisting of the vestibular nuclei and their central connections. The peripheral component has acceleration detectors (the semi-circular canals) and gravity detectors (the maculae of the saccule and utricle).

The vestibular end organ of each ear is formed by the three semi-circular canals set on different planes—the utricle, the saccule and the endolymphatic sac.

Each semi-circular canal has a bulbous end containing a crista ampullaris (Fig. 4.2) which responds to changes in angular acceleration. The inertia of the endolymph contained within the semi-circular canal causes a deflection of the sensory neuroepithelium of the crista, thereby altering the pattern of electrical impulses passing along the vestibular nerve.

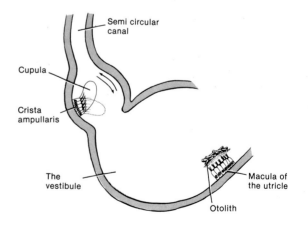

Fig. 4.2 Diagrammatic representation of the two types of vestibular receptors. The crista ampullaris deflects in response to angular acceleration. The macula of the utricle responds to linear acceleration, which induces a shearing movement between the otoliths and the cilia of the underlying hair cells.

The utricle contains a macula sensitive to changes in linear acceleration (Fig. 4.2). The exact function of the macula of the saccule is currently unclear. The endolymphatic sac appears to have an important role in the maintenance of normal endolymph homeostasis (pressure) and in the immune response of the inner ear.

5. Clinical examination of the ear

BASIC PRINCIPLES

Because the contents of the middle and inner ear are situated deeply within the temporal bone they are relatively inaccessible to direct examination. In the normal ear, only the auricle, external canal and tympanic membrane can be directly inspected. The middle ear contents can only be seen directly when a large perforation of the tympanic membrane is present. Nevertheless, as the only window into the middle ear, the appearance and behaviour of an intact tympanic membrane will give valuable information about possible disease within.

Since the middle ear cleft is both structurally and functionally related to the upper respiratory tract, an assessment of the ear is incomplete without a clinical examination of the upper airways, including the nose, nasopharynx, paranasal sinuses and oropharynx. Both ears must always be examined and, if disease is unilateral, it is generally advisable to examine the normal ear first, both to determine what may be normal for that particular patient and to avoid the possibility of cross-infection. Inspection of the good ear may also provide valuable clues to the status of the diseased organ.

HISTORY-TAKING

The successful diagnosis of any otological disorder depends on a sound clinical approach. The first step, as always, is to obtain a detailed history of the presenting complaint, paying particular attention to any previous ear disease or surgery that may have altered the normal architecture. Whilst otological symptoms are relatively few in number—e.g. itching, pain, discharge, hearing loss, tinnitus, dizziness and facial palsy—they are nevertheless key diagnostic pointers. Other important features such as, for example, a family history of ear discharge or hearing loss, exposure to toxins such as ototoxic drugs, noise exposure, prior disease, recent swimming or self-manipulation of the external ear canal will be brought out by asking direct questions.

TECHNIQUES OF EXAMINATION

Infants

Infants are most easily examined while they are sleeping. If awake, it is important to immobilize the head carefully but firmly and simultaneously to prevent sudden movements of the extremities. This can be readily achieved if the child is seated comfortably on the parent's lap and restrained with the side of the infant's head pinned against the parent's chest. If the child begins to cry, the ears must be examined without delay, since vigorous crying may cause a dilatation of the blood vessels supplying the tympanic membrane, producing an appearance which looks deceptively like that of an early acute otitis media. A particularly hyperactive or unco-operative infant can be wrapped in a blanket, a papoose-carrier or similar restraint and placed upon an examination table.

Pre-school children

Many pre-school children are apprehensive about a visit to the doctor, but it is usually possible to put a co-operative youngster at ease. It is advisable to remove one's white coat or head mirror prior to examining a child who is known to be particularly timid. A few moments playing a game with the otoscope will often gain a youngster's confidence and most children enjoy playing at blowing out the light. In order to minimize any fear of the unknown, the examiner must tell the child exactly what is to be done. A young child should not be asked for permission to examine the ears, since this may be refused. A better approach is to ask: 'which ear would you like me to look at first?' Interesting pictures strategically hung on the walls of the examination room can be used to engage a child's attention during examination. Gentleness, care and patience are essential when dealing with youngsters because if the examiner inflicts pain, it will be quite some time before confidence and co-operation can be re-established.

Adults

The examination of an adult is generally easier because the meatus will usually admit a larger speculum and therefore more light. The examiner can usually expect a reasonable degree of compliance, provided that the patient understands that the ear is to be inspected and care is taken to avoid unnecessary discomfort.

Hearing-handicapped patients

Most hearing-impaired patients are used to a regular examination of their ears, but it is nevertheless important to communicate with the patient on each occasion. This is especially important in those patients who have undergone previous ear surgery and may therefore have experienced pain or discomfort in the past.

THE OUTER EAR

A systematic examination of the ear always begins with a careful inspection of the auricle and the post-auricular skin. Any tenderness, obvious abnormalities, discharge or surgical scars should be carefully noted. In addition, there may be evidence of either a localized or a generalized skin disorder. At this stage, long hair can be controlled by draping it behind the auricle prior to further examination with the speculum or otoscope.

OTOSCOPY

The electric otoscope or auriscope is perfectly satisfactory for the majority of routine ear examinations. First the pinna should be gently palpated for tenderness and the entrance of the ear canal inspected (Fig. 5.1) for the presence of debris, pus, or local disease prior to the introduction of an appropriately sized speculum.

In order to obtain the widest field of view and at the same time admit the maximum amount of light into the depths of the ear canal, the largest speculum which can be comfortably inserted into the canal should be used. The following sizes of specula are most often used: for adults 4–6 mm and for children 3–4 mm; for infants a 2 mm diameter speculum may occasionally be necessary.

The speculum will enter more easily if the mobile outer cartilaginous part of the ear canal is straightened. In adults this is accomplished by gently lifting the pinna upward and backward (posterosuperiorly), and in young children by easing the pinna horizontally backward. It is quite possible to compress even a sizeable lesion such as an ulcer or a local polyp between the speculum and ear canal, and care should be taken to prevent the obvious being overlooked.

It is extremely important to hold the electric otoscope correctly, especially when examining young children who may suddenly move. The tip

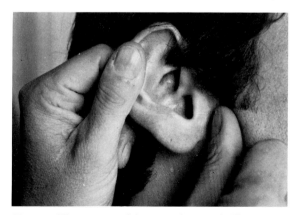

Fig. 5.1 The entrance of the external meatus is dilated and inspected by retracting the pinna posterosuperiorly in the left hand while counter-traction is applied with the right thumb in front of the tragus. For the left ear (see Fig. 5.6) the hand is hooked over the top of the pinna.

of the speculum should be manoeuvred under direct vision to rest gently in the lumen of the outer cartilaginous canal. The otoscope should be held in a manner so that even if the patient moves, the tip will not be impaled into the tender skin of the canal. This can be achieved if the instrument is held like a pencil (Fig. 5.2) between the thumb and the forefinger, with the ulnar aspect of the hand resting firmly but gently against the patient's cheek or neck. The bulb of the pneumatic attachment can then be conveniently held in the palm of the same hand. With this method, if the patient turns or moves suddenly, the otoscope will move in unison with the patient's head, and the possibility of injury to the ear canal or even the tympanic membrane will be avoided.

Due to the limited field of vision through even the largest speculum when magnification is used, only a portion of the tympanic membrane will be visible at any one time. The examiner is thus obliged to adjust both his or her line of sight and the position of the speculum within the canal to obtain a composite view of the entire tympanic membrane and deep meatus (Fig. 5.3).

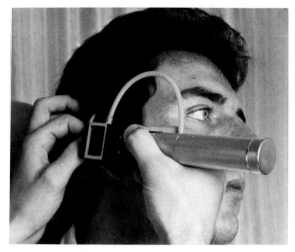

Fig. 5.2   While the pinna is retracted with the left hand, the tip of the otoscope is inserted into the external auditory canal. The otoscope is held in the right hand like a pen. The examiner's hand is resting firmly against the patient's cheek, to stabilize the otoscope. Notice that the rubber bulb of the Siegle attachment is held in the palm of the right hand.

Fig. 5.3   Because of the relatively narrow angle of view through the otoscope, the examiner must move both the otoscope and his or her eye in order to develop a composite view of the entire tympanic membrane and external auditory canal.

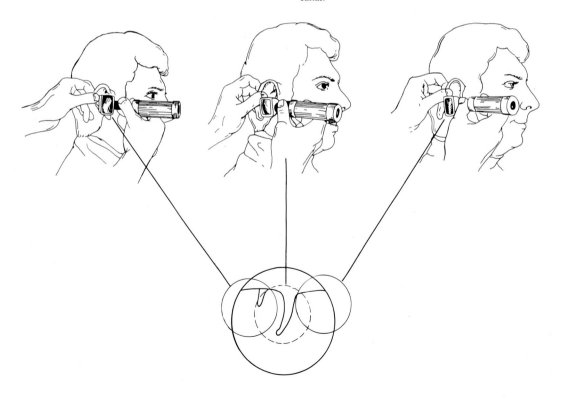

Furthermore, movements of the speculum within the canal alter the angle at which incident light strikes the tympanic membrane and produce a better appreciation of subtle changes from the normal. In contrast, by using a headlight or mirror and a large speculum held at arm's length, the entire tympanic membrane can normally be seen at a glance.

The examiner must be systematic while inspecting the ear, looking routinely at the malleus, attic area, all four quadrants of the pars tensa, the annulus and the deep external canal. A common error is to withdraw the otoscope before inspecting the skin of the superficial ear canal.

THE PNEUMATIC OTOSCOPE

Pneumatic otoscopy is a rapid and inexpensive diagnostic technique which is widely used by both otologists and primary care physicians to assess the tympanic membrane and middle ear. This technique involves observing the presence or absence of movement of the tympanic membrane by using the pneumatic attachment of the otoscope (Fig. 5.4). Valuable information about the pressure within the middle ear and the mobility of the tympanic membrane can be obtained by observing the relative movements of the pars tensa and the pars flaccida in response to the induced changes in the air pressure of the external canal. The mobility of the tympanic membrane can then be classified as normal, reduced, increased or absent.

This technique requires the use of a speculum large enough to fit snugly into the ear canal, in order to establish a closed air chamber between the canal and the interior of the otoscope head. Sofspecs (Welch Allyn) are extremely useful specula for pneumatic otoscopy because they have soft, pliable tips which fit snugly into the external canal and produce an excellent air seal.

The pressure of the air within the canal can then be increased by gently squeezing the small valveless rubber bulb of the pneumatic attachment. Pneumatic otoscopy should be performed gently, and the patient should be warned beforehand that a feeling of pressure in the ear will be experienced and that a blowing noise may be heard; otherwise children, and indeed some adults, may be startled. When the tympanic membrane and the pressure within the

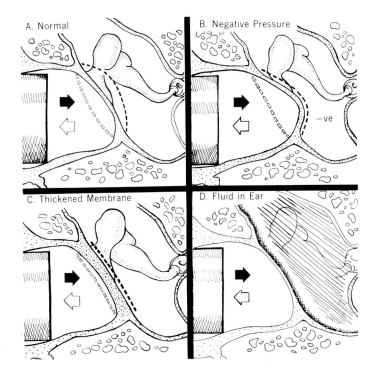

Fig. 5.4 In the normal ear (**A**) the tympanic membrane demonstrates a crisp inward movement as positive pressure is applied and a similar outward movement as the pressure is released. Where there is negative pressure (**B**) within the middle ear the tympanic membrane is retracted and little inward movement is seen with positive pressure, although some outward movement can still be observed as the pressure is released. With a thickened tympanic membrane (**C**), limited movement to both positive and negative pressure is usually observed. If the middle ear is filled with fluid (**D**), there is usually a total absence of tympanic membrane movement. (After J. Coulter.)

middle ear (intratympanic pressure) are normal the tympanic membrane will show a crisp inward movement as the pressure within the otoscope head is increased by squeezing the rubber bulb. When the rubber bulb is released, and the pressure within the canal rapidly returns to normal, the tympanic membrane will then snap crisply outwards.

If the air pressure within the middle ear is negative, due to an obstructed eustachian tube, the tympanic membrane will only move sluggishly. Fluid within the middle ear will usually result in a severe decrease or even a total absence of mobility. When the tympanic membrane is immobile, the only movement observed may be a slight outward displacement of the soft and compressible outer cartilaginous external canal. The pneumatic otoscope may also be useful in distinguishing between a thin, atrophic, intact tympanic membrane plastered to the promontory, which may be made to move, and a large perforation which will not move. This simple clinical procedure provides an easy and inexpensive method of determining tympanic membrane mobility and is of invaluable assistance in the early diagnosis and recognition of many middle ear disorders.

TRADITIONAL SPECULUM EXAMINATION OF THE EAR

Either reflected (head mirror) or direct (headlight) illumination can be used for a speculum examination. Traditionally, otolaryngologists have used a reflected source of light to examine the ear. Illumination from a powerful tungsten or halogen lamp (100 W) placed beside the patient is reflected into the ear canal by means of a head mirror (Figs 5.5 and 5.6). The head mirror is perforated to allow the examiner to look through the central hole, thereby maintaining coaxial, parallax-free, binocular vision. The mirror should also be concave, in order to concentrate and focus the light at a distance of about 17 cm.

Most examiners in Canada and Europe prefer to position the head mirror over the dominant (right) eye and place the source of illumination on their right-hand side, slightly above and behind the patient. In the USA it is customary to position the mirror over the left or non-dominant eye, with the source of illumination on the examiner's left, so that if instruments are used the operating hand does not obstruct the beam of light.

A certain amount of practice is needed to adjust the head mirror so that the light is reflected and concentrated into the speculum. Initially, alignment of the head mirror is facilitated if the eye which is not behind the mirror is first closed. With the mirror correctly positioned, the examiner can achieve an

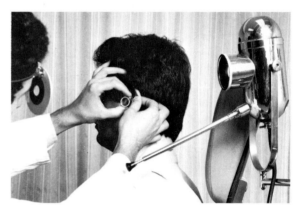

Fig. 5.5 Using a head mirror and a bull's-eye lamp, the examiner is inserting a speculum into the external auditory canal. The pinna is retracted between the thumb and index finger of the right hand and the speculum held between the thumb and middle finger of the left hand.

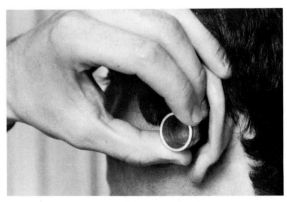

Fig. 5.6 Once the speculum has been inserted into the external canal it can be held with one hand, leaving the other free for instrumentation. The speculum is held between the thumb and index finger of the hand while the pinna is retracted between the middle and ring fingers.

unobstructed view down the speculum with both eyes and enjoy stereoscopic vision. The head mirror is not recommended for occasional otoscopists unless they have had substantial practice with this technique.

The portable electric headlight is a useful alternative to the head mirror as a source of illumination. Electric headlights can be powered either from the a.c. (mains) supply via a voltage stepdown transformer or from a portable battery pack. The electric headlight is generally more convenient than a head mirror for domiciliary or bedside examinations. Furthermore, headlights are somewhat easier to use because the beam of light remains in a fixed position relative to the examiner and is less affected by movements of the patient. The disadvantage is that they do not provide parallax-free illumination.

If magnification is required during speculum examination of the ear canal and tympanic membrane, a Stierlen's magnifying loupe can be clipped over the end of the speculum. This loupe incorporates a semi-circular lens which allows the passage of instruments into the ear canal.

The addition of a Siegle otoscopic attachment (Fig. 5.7) to the speculum will allow an assessment of tympanic membrane mobility to be made under direct magnified vision (pneumatic otoscopy). This traditional device consists of a circular magnifying lens obliquely set in a holder which incorporates a nipple, to which a valveless rubber bulb can be attached. Squeezing the bulb induces alterations of air pressure within the external canal, and if the middle ear cleft is normally aerated, an intact tympanic membrane can be made to move quite freely.

The Siegle otoscope should be positioned so that the magnifying lens is angled upwards (Fig. 5.8). In this way, the lens is automatically set at the correct angle to prevent reflection of light from the surface of the magnifying lens back into the examiner's eye, and a satisfactory view of the tympanic membrane can be obtained.

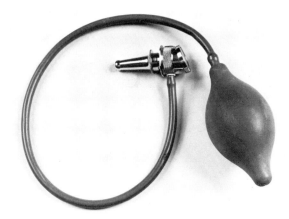

Fig. 5.7 The Siegle pneumatic otoscope. Notice the valveless rubber bulb attached to a small nipple. The glass magnifying lens which encloses the system is angled to prevent light reflecting back into the examiner's eye.

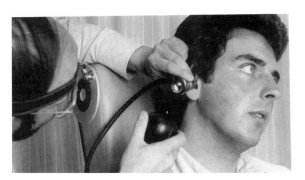

Fig. 5.8 The Siegle otoscope is positioned with the magnifying lens angled upwards, thereby placing the angled lens in the correct position to prevent reflection of light back into the examiner's eyes. Variations in the air pressure in the external canal are induced by gently squeezing and releasing the rubber bulb.

CERUMEN

The ear canal is frequently occluded by wax and debris, which must be completely removed if the entire tympanic membrane is to be seen and a proper otoscopic examination accomplished. This is of fundamental importance, since many ear disorders can only be diagnosed accurately if key physical signs are recognized.

Cerumen (ear wax) is an accumulation of sebum and secretions from the ceruminous glands, mixed with keratin desquamated from the skin of the external canal. The ceruminous glands are modified sweat glands located in the hair-bearing outer third of the external auditory canal. Cerumen varies widely in both colour and consistency and can range from golden-yellow flakes (Fig. 5.9) to sticky brownish material (Fig. 5.10) or hard dark concretions (Fig. 5.11). In most Orientals, the ceruminous glands appear to be different, and the cerumen appears dry, golden-yellow in colour and rather flaky ('rice-bran wax'; Fig. 5.12).

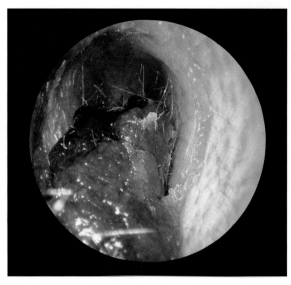

Fig. 5.10   Soft brown sticky wax is seen filling the inferior half of the external canal.

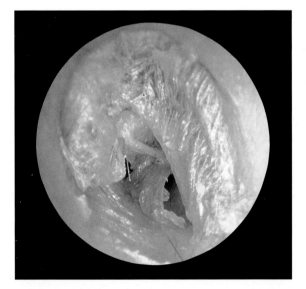

Fig. 5.9   A thin film of golden-yellow wax almost completely occludes the entrance of the external canal.

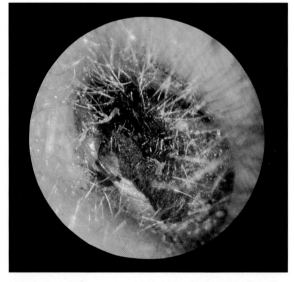

Fig. 5.11   The entire external canal is filled with a dark, hard plug of wax.

Wax and keratin debris may be intermixed in some ears (Fig. 5.13). This type of plug may sometimes be quite firmly attached to the underlying skin (Fig. 5.14). Patients who use cotton-tipped applicators to clean their ears frequently push the wax into the deep meatus until it lies directly against the tympanic membrane (Fig. 5.15). Sometimes quite large

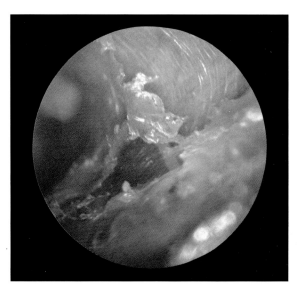

Fig. 5.14 The same patient as illustrated in Figure 5.13 after removal of the wax and keratin debris. Notice how the keratin has been closely adherent to the underlying canal skin. A small haematoma has been produced by the trauma of separating the keratin from the underlying skin.

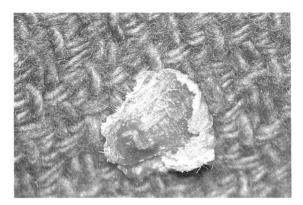

Fig. 5.12 Notice the dry, golden-yellow Oriental 'rice-bran' type wax.

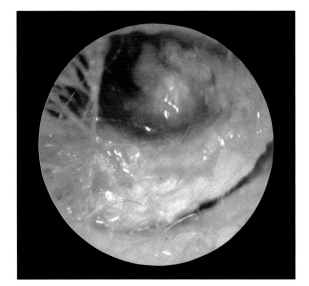

Fig. 5.13 In this patient both wax and desquamated skin (keratin) are seen, filling the external canal. The keratin is often adherent to the underlying skin.

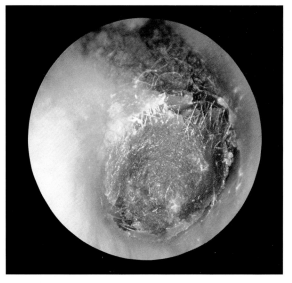

Fig. 5.15 A mixture of wax and hair has been pushed into the deep meatus by the insertion of a cotton-tipped applicator and is lying up against the tympanic membrane.

plugs of wax filling the entire external canal will be removed (Figs 5.16 and 5.17).

Wax can be removed by syringing or by instrumentation (curettage or suction) under direct vision. When the introduction of water into the ear is contraindicated (e.g. in cases of known or suspected tympanic membrane perforation, after recent trauma or when a history of recent inflammatory ear disease has been obtained), then instrumentation becomes the preferred method of cleaning the ear, since the entry of water into the middle ear frequently leads to infection.

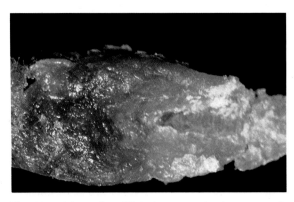

Fig. 5.16 A large plug of light-brown wax has been removed from the external canal.

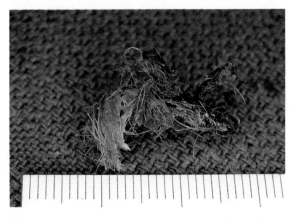

Fig. 5.17 In this patient the entire meatus was filled with this mixture of hair and cerumen.

Aural syringing

An ear should never be syringed unless the tympanic membrane is known to be normal. If syringing is indicated, certain technical details are important. Syringing is best carried out under direct vision, using either a head mirror or a headlight to provide sufficient illumination.

When using a metal aural syringe, care should be taken to ensure that the plunger moves freely, without sticking, and that the nozzle is securely screwed into place. If the nozzle is not firmly attached to the barrel of the syringe it could be propelled into the ear during forceful syringing, causing serious damage to the tympanic membrane and ossicles. The aural syringe should be dismantled and cleaned periodically and the piston lubricated with glycerine or petroleum jelly to prevent sticking and wear.

Tap water at body temperature (37°C) is satisfactory for ear syringing. When the syringe has been filled with water, it should be held vertically, nozzle up and all air expressed. This is to prevent syringing with a mixture of water and bubbles, which is extremely noisy and uncomfortable for the patient, as well as to allow the direct transmission of the force on the plunger to the stream of water, because if there is a collection of air within the syringe it will act as a buffer as it is compressed and the stream of water will not have sufficient force to wash out the cerumen. Most otolaryngologists believe that if water that is appreciably warmer or cooler than normal body temperature (37°C) is used for syringing, then a caloric response (thermal stimulation of the inner ear) may be produced and the patient can experience an unpleasant transient dizziness. However, one of the authors of this book (MH) routinely uses warmer water (44°C) for syringing because the warmer water seems to break up the cerumen plug more efficiently. To date the use of water at this temperature has not produced a caloric response.

The patient should be seated comfortably and draped with a plastic sheet covered by an absorbent towel to protect the clothing. A kidney basin, which the patient holds tightly against the side of the neck, is placed under the ear to catch the effluent.

The ear canal is straightened by gently

retracting the pinna up and backwards in adults, and horizontally backwards in children. The nozzle of the syringe is then gently introduced into the entrance of the external canal *under direct vision* and positioned so that the stream of water is directed at the roof of the canal (Fig. 5.18). In most instances, the wax will fragment easily in the stream of warm water and emerge without difficulty.

If the canal is occluded by a firm plug, the aim is then to insinuate the water between the tympanic membrane and the wax, thereby pushing or flushing out the plug. This is achieved by angling the nozzle up and backwards; if the water is squirted straight into the canal it will simply push the wax in more deeply (Fig. 5.19).

A piece of absorbent tissue or cotton wool held to the ear while the bowl is being emptied will prevent the accidental wetting of the patient's neck and clothing. After all debris has been removed, the external canal is thoroughly dried with cotton wool (Fig. 5.20) and carefully inspected. Following ear syringing, the tympanic membrane frequently appears pink and dilatation of the tympanic blood vessels can be seen. If any inadvertent trauma of the skin lining has occurred, the patient should simply be instructed to keep the skin dry to prevent the development of infection until the area has healed.

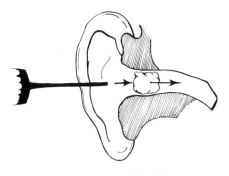

INCORRECT

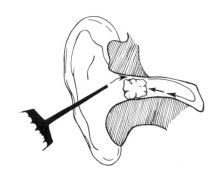

CORRECT

Fig. 5.19 If the jet of water from the aural syringe is directed at the wax plug, it will be pushed deeper into the canal (top). The tip of the syringe should be angled so that the jet of water passes above the wax plug into the deep canal, thereby forcing the plug of cerumen outwards (bottom).

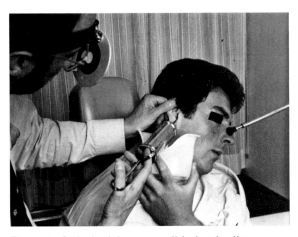

Fig. 5.18 Syringing is best accomplished under direct vision. Notice that the syringe is angled into the posterosuperior quadrant. This is facilitated by having the patient tilt the head away from the examiner.

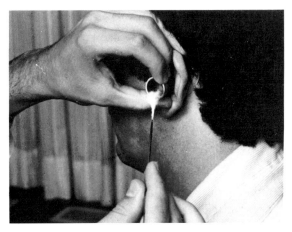

Fig. 5.20 The external canal can be dried with cotton wool under direct vision using a speculum.

Wax removal by instrumentation

In the hands of a skilled operator, soft wax may be aspirated using a large suction tip (Fig. 5.21). Firm wax can be removed safely using a blunt hook or ring-ended probe. Adequate illumination (e.g. a headlight or head mirror), an unobstructed view of the external canal and manual dexterity are essential if trauma to the delicate canal-wall skin or middle ear structures is to be avoided. Furthermore, successful instrumentation requires a co-operative patient who is capable of sitting still. In difficult cases it may be necessary to resort to the use of a binocular operating microscope to clean the ear canal safely and thoroughly.

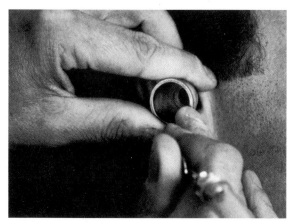

Fig. 5.21 Soft wax and purulent debris can frequently be removed under direct vision using a speculum. Note how the examiner's right little finger rests against the patient's cheek, in order to stabilize the hand holding the suction tube.

Ceruminolytics

If syringing or instrumentation does not readily dislodge a plug of wax, further attempts at removal are likely to cause unnecessary trauma. The patient is then advised to instil a bland ceruminolytic into the ear canal for 5 days before returning. The best ceruminolytic is a 20–30% solution of sodium bicarbonate in distilled water. Cerumen is not significantly softened or dissolved by oily or organic solutions. Many proprietary ceruminolytics contain turpentine or other skin irritants and should not be used because these solutions are ineffective and may cause a severe contact dermatitis of the external canal.

Purulent debris

If purulent debris is found in the ear canal, a swab should be taken for laboratory culture (both for bacteria and fungi) and sensitivity testing before proceeding to clean the ear, using suction or dry mopping with a cotton wool-tipped probe. The presence of purulent debris in the canal is generally a contraindication to aural syringing.

Mastoid cavities

To prevent excessive accumulation of wax and debris and the development of underlying infection, a mastoid or fenestration cavity should be cleaned every 6–12 months. If the meatus is small or there is a high facial ridge (see Chapter 9), this may be difficult and is best left to an experienced otologist. In these patients care must be exercised, since the architecture of the cavity may expose the facial nerve, the stapes footplate or the lateral semi-circular canal to possible injury during manipulation.

THE FISTULA TEST

The fistula test is accomplished by inducing pronounced variations in the air pressure within the external canal, and can be simply carried out either by rapidly and repeatedly compressing the bulb of the pneumatic attachment to the otoscope or by repeatedly pressing on the tragal cartilage with the index finger.

If an abnormal communication exists between the external auditory canal and the membranous labyrinth, giddiness (vertigo) or, in more extensive cases, nystagmus will be elicited. This abnormal communication is generally situated in the lateral semi-circular canal. A positive fistula sign denotes not only an abnormal opening into the bony labyrinth but also the presence of a functioning vestibular end organ.

The fistula test should be performed routinely on any patient with a history of dizziness in whom erosion of the bony labyrinth by infection, cholesteatoma or tumour is suspected. It should also be carried out when a cholesteatoma is discovered clinically in an otherwise asymptomatic patient.

CLINICAL TESTS OF EUSTACHIAN TUBE FUNCTION

Aeration of the middle ear cleft is dependent upon a normally functioning eustachian tube. Since most disorders affecting the middle ear can be attributed to eustachian tube dysfunction, an examination of the ear is incomplete without an inspection of the nasopharynx and a functional assessment of the eustachian tube. A healthy eustachian tube is normally closed, and only opens during swallowing and yawning.

Toynbee's manoeuvre

The patency of the eustachian tube during normal swallowing can be determined in some individuals by observing the tympanic membrane while the patient swallows with the nose pinched firmly closed. If the eustachian tube opens during swallowing, a simultaneous inward movement of the tympanic membrane may be seen.

Valsalva manoeuvre (autoinflation)

The ability of the eustachian tube to open when the pressure in the nasopharynx is raised can be assessed by instructing the patient forcefully to blow air into the nose with the mouth closed and with the external nares tightly pinched between the thumb and forefinger. If the patient's eustachian tube opens during this manoeuvre, the tympanic membrane will 'pop' or bulge outwards as air enters the middle ear. This entry of air into the middle ear can actually be heard if the patient's ear is connected to the examiner's ear by means of a Toynbee listening tube.

Approximately 30% of normal subjects are unable to autoinflate the middle ear successfully, so that even if the tympanic membrane appears immobile, the examiner must not automatically assume that the eustachian tube is abnormal.

Abnormal eustachian tube patency (patulous tube)

In some instances, the eustachian tube may be abnormally patent (open) and can be responsible for a number of auditory symptoms including fluttering tinnitus, autophonia, reverberation or 'blockage'. In these individuals, the tympanic membrane moves with nasal respiration. This phenomenon can be demonstrated by observing the tympanic membrane while the patient inhales and exhales forcefully through the nose whilst occluding the opposite nostril.

ADDITIONAL INVESTIGATIONS

After a detailed history has been taken and a full clinical examination of the ear has been completed, the examiner is in a position to select those appropriate tests of auditory and vestibular function which will lead to an accurate diagnosis. A detailed discussion and description of these tests is beyond the scope of this text, but can be found in any standard textbook of otology; some are listed in the bibliography.

Tuning fork tests

The traditional tuning fork tests still remain simple and essential preliminary tests in the diagnosis of hearing loss.

The Rinne test

When the sound-conducting mechanism of the inner ear is normal, the usual route of sound transmission (air conduction) is more efficient and this air-conducted sound will be perceived by the patient to be louder than that transmitted by bone conduction (*positive Rinne*).

The sound from a vibrating tuning fork placed near the entrance of the external auditory meatus is conducted via the normal middle ear mechanism to the cochlea. This air conduction hearing is a measure of both the cochlear reserve and the middle ear sound-conducting mechanism. The sound from a vibrating tuning fork placed on the mastoid process is conducted directly to the cochlea, bypassing the normal middle ear mechanism. This bone conduction hearing is a measure of cochlear function. Thus, diminished hearing by bone conduction indicates a sensorineural or perceptive deafness. In the presence of a conductive hearing loss, air conduction sound is impeded from reaching the cochlea, whereas bone conduction sound passes with ease and may appear louder.

In the Rinne test, the patient is asked to compare the loudness of a tuning fork held near the entrance of the external auditory canal—air conduction (Fig. 5.22)—with the loudness of the fork placed on the lateral aspect of the mastoid process—bone conduction (Fig. 5.23). If the tuning fork is perceived as being louder by air conduction than by bone conduction, *the Rinne is described as positive*. This indicates a normal sound-conducting mechanism within the middle ear. If the tuning fork is heard louder by bone conduction than by air conduction, *the Rinne is described as negative*, indicating a conductive hearing loss.

False negative Rinne.   Where there is a total or severe sensorineural hearing loss in one ear, the patient may hear the tuning fork when it is placed over the mastoid process of that ear. In this case, the sound of the tuning fork is being transmitted across the skull by bone conduction and perceived by the patient's good ear. This is termed a *false negative Rinne*.

A Bárány noise box or other source of masking noise should be used to confirm the diagnosis of a severe or total sensorineural hearing loss in one ear. The mechanical sound produced by the box is used to mask the good ear, thus preventing a false negative Rinne occurring.

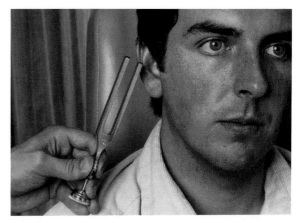

Fig. 5.22   The Rinne test assessing air conduction.

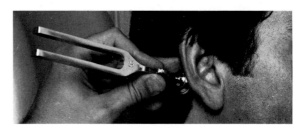

Fig. 5.23   The Rinne test assessing bone conduction.

The Weber test

The second important diagnostic tuning fork test is the Weber test (Fig. 5.24). This test determines whether monaural impairment is of conductive or neural origin by comparing the bone conduction of both ears. The sound stimulus from the base of the tuning fork on the top of the skull reaches both temporal bones by bone conduction at the same time and with the same intensity. If the sound-conducting mechanism of the middle ear is normal, then the loudness of the sound will be heard in the ear which has the better cochlea (will be lateralized to the better ear).

If the sound-conducting mechanism of the ear is not normal, then the tuning fork will be perceived as being louder in that ear (will be lateralized to the poorer ear).

These tuning fork tests are summarized in Figure 5.25.

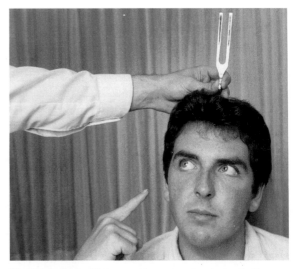

Fig. 5.24   In the Weber test the patient is asked to indicate in which ear the sound is heard.

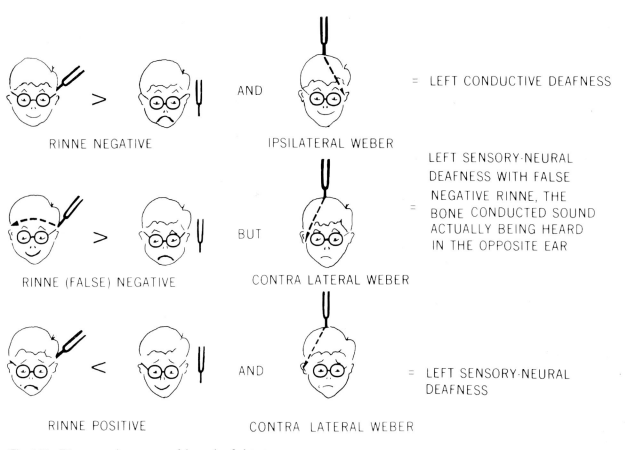

Fig. 5.25 Diagrammatic summary of the tuning fork tests.

6. Diseases of the pinna

INTRODUCTION

The external ear consists of the pinna, the external auditory canal and the outermost layer of the tympanic membrane. The pinna (Latin for feather) or external auricle (from the Latin *auricula*, the diminutive of *auris*, ear) is a convoluted and flattened funnel-shaped appendage whose shape is determined by the underlying flexible elastic auricular cartilage. The auricular cartilage is contiguous with the cartilage of the outer portion of the external auditory canal. In the human, the pinna plays only a rudimentary function in the amplification and localization of sound, whereas in lower mammals such as the bat and the dog this function is highly developed.

In addition to its auditory function, the folds and convolutions of the pinna provide some protection by shielding the external canal from direct trauma. As the pinna is attached to the side of the head in a relatively exposed position, it is subject both to local trauma and to the immediate and delayed effects of solar radiation.

The pinna is formed in the embryo by the coalescence of six tiny hillocks or tubercles, located on the dorsal end of the first (mandibular) and second (hyoid) branchial arches. There is a wide variation in the size and shape of the normal auricle, and minor developmental abnormalities are often found.

A severe congenital malformation of the pinna may, however, be associated with an abnormality of the middle or inner ear, and should alert the examiner to the possibility of an underlying hearing loss. Although most congenital malformations are genetic in origin, exposure of the fetus to drugs or infection can result in an abnormality in the position or shape of the pinna.

Darwin's tubercle

Darwin's tubercle (Fig. 6.1) is a small cartilaginous protuberance, most commonly located along the concave edge of the posterosuperior margin of the helix, which projects anteriorly. Less commonly (Fig. 6.2), Darwin's tubercle projects posteriorly.

This atavistic remnant represents the apex of the anthropoid ear and suggests a common ancestry between man and ape, and for this reason it is called Darwin's tubercle. Darwin's tubercles are inherited by means of an autosomal dominant gene which has a variable expressivity. These tubercles have no clinical significance.

CONGENITAL MALFORMATIONS AND DISEASES OF THE EAR

As the external, middle and inner ears differ in both their embryological origins and times of development, there is a wide variation in the types of abnormality that can be encountered. Patients may be seen who have an absent auricle and external auditory canal and yet have only a minimal deformity of the middle ear and a normal inner ear. By contrast, some children may have a normal or almost normal external ear and a severe congenital malformation of the underlying middle and inner ears.

Congenital abnormalities of the ear may be unilateral or bilateral and of course may be associated with congenital malformations elsewhere in the body. These deformities may be the result of a genetic defect, the result of a viral infection or of exposure to ototoxic drugs during the first trimester.

Atresia of the pinna and external canal

Absence or partial maldevelopment of the pinna is frequently associated with abnormalities of the external auditory canal and underlying middle ear; the inner ear in these patients is usually normal. In the patient shown in Figure 6.3 the inferior half of the conchal bowl is not fully developed, giving the ear a feline appearance. The small pit seen in the concha ended blindly a short distance medially. This failure in the development of the external auditory meatus was

associated with a deformity of the middle ear and ossicles. In the patient shown in Figure. 6.4 there is no opening for the external canal (complete meatal atresia).

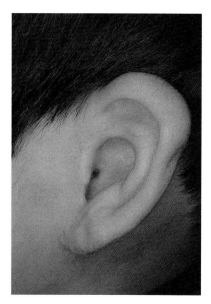

Fig. 6.3   Partial atresia.

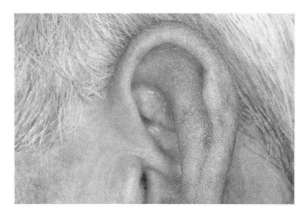

Fig. 6.1   Common Darwin's tubercle.

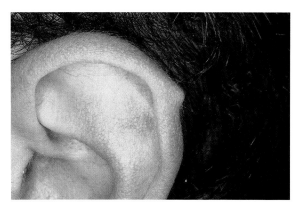

Fig. 6.2   Uncommon Darwin's tubercle projecting posteriorly.

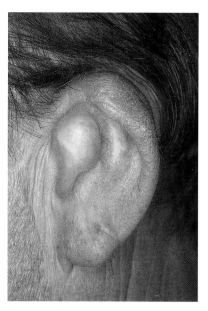

Fig. 6.4   Congenital atresia of the external canal.

Microtia (Fig. 6.5)

The term *microtia* is used when there is gross hypoplasia of the pinna with a blind or absent external auditory canal. Microtia encompasses a wide spectrum of severe malformations, ranging from a mere nubbin of tissue on the side of the head which has no recognizable features to a formed auricular appendage that is obviously deformed and smaller than normal. Microtia is typically bilateral, although the degree of the deformity may be different on the two sides.

Children born with microtia should have their hearing tested soon after birth, and if a hearing loss is present, should be fitted with a hearing aid as quickly as possible.

A computerized tomography scan should be done to determine if the middle ear structures are sufficiently normal for middle ear reconstructive surgery to be successful. Because this type of surgery is technically difficult and potentially hazardous to both the inner ear and the facial nerve, it should only be performed by an otologist who is experienced in operating on this type of patient. If the microtia is unilateral, middle ear reconstructive surgery is generally not recommended. Reconstructive surgery may also be performed to rebuild the pinna into a more cosmetically normal structure.

Outstanding ears (bat ears)

Outstanding, protruding or bat ears are the commonest cosmetic deformity of the pinna. Outstanding ears are inherited by means of an autosomal dominant gene which has complete penetrance but a variable expressivity. Clinically the angle between the auricle and the side of the head is greater than normal and the auricle protrudes anteriorly (Fig. 6.6). In addition there may be a poorly formed antihelical fold or excessive tissue, usually in the conchal or the triangular fossae, giving the ear a cupped appearance (Fig. 6.7).

While outstanding ears are asymptomatic, once children with such ears find that they are the object of ridicule by their peers, the emotional discomfort is often such that otoplasty is required to remove the source of their anxiety. The ideal time for such surgery is generally between 4 and 6 years of age.

Otoplasty consists of the excision of an elliptical area of the post-auricular skin combined with releasing incisions in the posterior portion of the auricular cartilage to weaken its outwardly projecting springiness and to create a strong and well defined antihelix. This

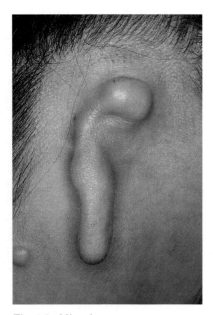

Fig. 6.5   Microtia.

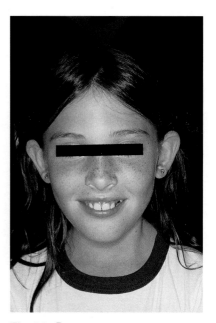

Fig. 6.6   Bat ears.

operation requires some skill, not only to produce a cosmetically satisfactory result, but also to ensure that the two sides look alike.

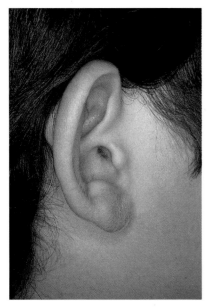

Fig. 6.7   Bat ears (cupped appearance).

Pre-auricular tags

Pre-auricular tags (Fig. 6.8) are tiny raised nubbins of skin located along the anterior border of the ear in front of the tragus. Pre-auricular tags are soft, mobile and filled with soft tissue.

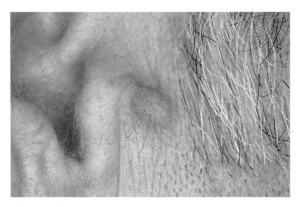

Fig. 6.8   Pre-auricular tag.

Accessory auricles (Fig. 6.9)

Accessory auricles differ from pre-auricular tags in that they contain a small island of cartilage.

These accessory auricles are believed to represent the remnant of one of the embryological hillocks. While both pre-auricular tags and accessory auricles have no clinical significance, they may be excised for cosmetic reasons.

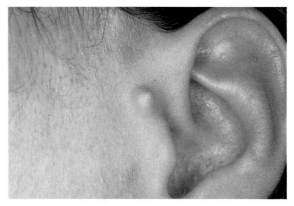

Fig. 6.9   Accessory auricle.

Pre-auricular pits, sinuses, and fistulas

Defective closure of the first branchial cleft or a failure in the fusion of the primitive ear hillocks may result in the formation of a small pit, sinus, or fistula related to the external ear. This deformity may vary from a small dimple (pre-auricular pit; Fig. 6.10) to a larger sinus

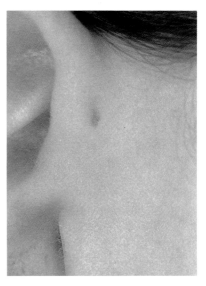

Fig. 6.10   Pre-auricular pit.

(pre-auricular sinus; Fig. 6.11). Pre-auricular pits and sinuses may become infected (Figs 6.12 and 6.13), and if they do, the infection frequently recurs.

Rarely, a pre-auricular fistula will be found as an abnormal communication between the skin of the face or neck and the external auditory canal (collaural fistula).

A pre-auricular sinus or fistula may be intimately related to the facial nerve or its branches, and the excision of these lesions should be left to an experienced surgeon.

Pre-auricular pit

Pre-auricular pits are shallow invaginations in the skin of the face which are located just in front of the anterior border of the anterior crus of the helix. A cheesy discharge of desquamated keratin debris is sometimes encountered.

Pre-auricular pits are inherited by means of an autosomal dominant gene with incomplete penetrance and are most commonly seen in orientals, occurring in 10–14% of the population, and in blacks (5%). They are most commonly unilateral (75%).

Pre-auricular sinus

If the invagination in front of the ear is relatively deep then the term pre-auricular sinus is more appropriate. A pre-auricular sinus (Fig. 6.11) is deeper than a pit and lined with a stratified squamous keratinizing epithelium. Gentle sounding with a small lacrimal duct probe can be used to establish the depth of the pre-auricular depression and distinguish a pre-auricular pit from a pre-auricular sinus. Pre-auricular sinuses are usually asymptomatic until they become infected (Figs 6.12, 6.13).

Infected pre-auricular sinus

If pathogenic bacteria enter the opening of a pre-auricular sinus, then the tract may become infected. If the tract of an infected pre-auricular sinus is patent, then a milky purulent material will be seen oozing on to the skin surface (Fig. 6.12). If, however, the opening of the pre-auricular sinus is occluded, a pre-auricular

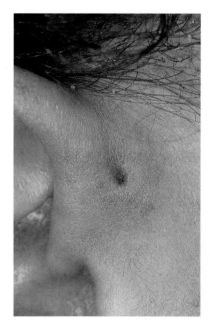

Fig. 6.11   Pre-auricular sinus.

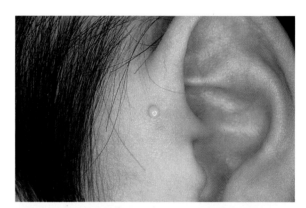

Fig. 6.12   Infected pre-auricular sinus.

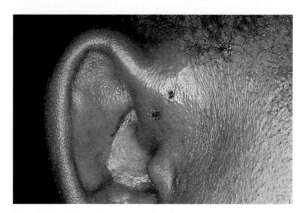

Fig. 6.13   Infected pre-auricular sinus.

abscess may then form. Pain, tenderness and swelling in front of the anterior border of the helix suggests the presence of a pre-auricular abscess (Fig. 6.13). The commonest infecting organisms are the Gram-positive anaerobic cocci, e.g. *Peptococcus*, *Peptostreptococcus* and *Bacteroides*. Once a pre-auricular sinus has become infected, there is a strong likelihood of recurrent infections.

The definitive treatment requires a complete excision of the entire sinus tract. Great care must be taken during the excision of a pre-auricular sinus because these sinuses may extend quite deeply and may be closely related to the branches of the facial nerve.

Hairy tragus (Fig. 6.14)

With ageing, coarse hairs may appear on the tragus of some males. This is a form of secondary sexual characteristic which has been called the hairy tragus. It is interesting to note that the Greek word *tragus* (goat) alludes to these hairs which bear a fancied resemblance to the beard of a goat.

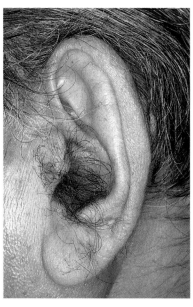

Fig. 6.14   Hairy tragus.

Hairy pinna (Fig 6.15)

In some individuals, with age, coarse hairs may appear on the lower portions of the helix. This type of ear is referred to as a hairy pinna. Hairy pinna occurs only in males, and is a Y-linked or holandric trait. The expression of this Y-linked trait increases with age, and there is an almost complete expression by the age of 60. Hairy pinna is most commonly encountered in the male population of India.

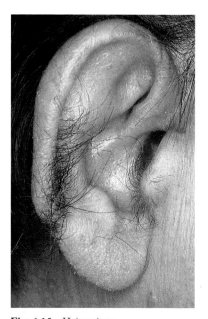

Fig. 6.15   Hairy pinna.

Traumatic seroma (othaematoma) (Fig. 6.16)

Acute or chronic friction which irritates the underlying perichondrium may result in the formation of a subperichondral serous or serosanguinous effusion. A seroma should be aseptically aspirated in order to prevent devitalization and subsequent necrosis of the underlying cartilage. After the fluid has been aspirated, the perichondrium should be gently compressed on to the cartilage by an inert (stainless steel or monofilament nylon) mattress suture using a button on either side of the pinna to maintain gentle pressure for 10–14 days (Fig. 6.17).

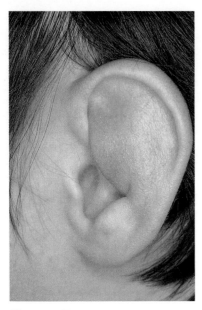

Fig. 6.16   Traumatic seroma.

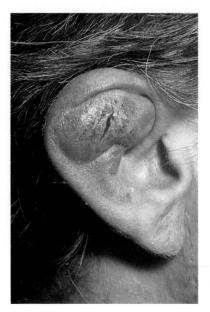

Fig. 6.18   Haematoma.

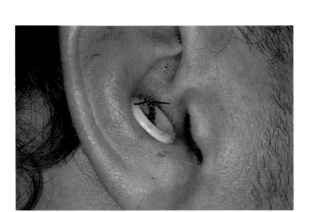

Fig. 6.17   Seroma after drainage.

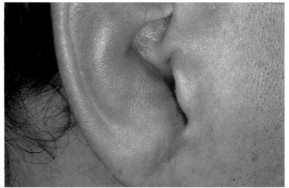

Fig. 6.19   Haematoma.

Haematoma

Haematomas of the auricle are usually the result of blunt trauma such as boxing, rugger and those other physical activities in which the skin of the pinna is exposed to twisting or shearing forces. The skin of the lateral surface of the auricle is tightly attached to the underlying perichondrium, and the small blood vessels that lie between the perichondrium and the underlying auricular cartilage are easily ruptured by a shearing force. Once a vessel is torn, blood will leak into the subperichondrial plane (between the perichondrium and the cartilage), thereby elevating the perichondrium from the underlying cartilage. This subperichondrial haematoma forms a soft blue or purple bulge that balloons the skin over the lateral surface of the pinna and distorts its normal sharp contours (Figs 6.18 and 6.19).

If the haematoma is not removed, then the subperichondrial collection of blood will persist, depriving the underlying cartilage of its critical perichondrial nourishment, thereby producing an avascular necrosis of the involved cartilage. A

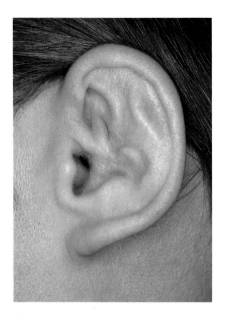

Fig. 6.20   Cauliflower ear.

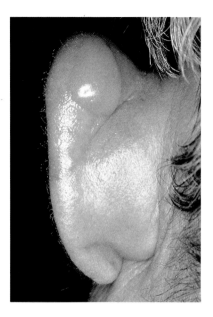

Fig. 6.21   Frostbite.

late sequela is the organization of the haematoma by the ingrowth of fibrous tissue and the development of a cauliflower ear (Fig. 6.20).

A simple aspiration of the haematoma is not sufficient as it will almost always recur. The entire collection of blood should be aspirated under sterile conditions and the skin held down against the underlying cartilage by through and through sutures (Fig. 6.17) as discussed in the treatment of traumatic seroma. Antibiotic coverage should be provided to prevent the development of acute perichondritis and subsequent cartilage necrosis.

Cauliflower ear

Repeated episodes of blunt trauma to the pinna, e.g. after boxing, rugby, football etc., which produce areas of subperichondrial separation or haemorrhage will cause necrosis and softening of the underlying auricular cartilage. The fibrosis that develops during the healing of these damaged areas usually results in both thickening and deformity of the lateral surface of the pinna. This type of post-traumatic deformity is called a cauliflower ear (Fig. 6.20). This patient was a boxer.

Frostbite (Fig. 6.21)

The pinna, by virtue of its exposed location, presents a large surface area in relation to its blood supply and is consequently subject to damage from extreme cold. The effect of cold temperature is increased by exposure to wind and by the presence of moisture on the exposed skin. Exposure to very low temperatures causes a severe and prolonged vasoconstriction of the capillary walls, resulting in damage to these walls. The anaesthesia which occurs in those areas of the skin exposed to the cold allows a significant amount of damage to occur 'silently' without the patient's knowledge.

Frostbite is usually characterized by a reddish or blue discoloration of the pinna, often accompanied by serum-filled blisters which resemble a second-degree burn (Fig. 6.21). The superior third of the pinna is most commonly affected by frostbite.

A frostbitten ear should be gradually rewarmed and protected by a sterile dressing in order to prevent the development of secondary infection. Early surgical debridement is best avoided, since it may take several months for the delineation between viable and dead tissue to occur.

Late calcification of the auricular cartilage following frostbite

Delayed dystrophic calcification or heterotopic calcification of the underlying auricular cartilage may develop years after the initial frostbite. When this occurs, the pinna is bony and hard to palpation. A radiograph of the pinna will reveal radiodense areas of calcification in the auricular cartilage (Fig. 6.22).

Impetigo

The superficial layers of the epidermis may become infected with *Staphylococcus aureus* or *Streptococcus pyogenes* (Fig. 6.23). The initial lesion consists of an infected vesicle or pustule that ruptures and dries to produce the typical yellowish crusts. Both the pustules and the crusts contain viable bacteria and are highly contagious. Macerated and moist skin is particularly susceptible to bacterial infections. This condition is surprisingly painless and the most common symptom is the presence of the crusty scabs and local itching. Treatment consists of the application of a topical cream containing an

antibiotic which is effective against the causative organisms, e.g. Bactroban.

Acute perichondritis (Fig. 6.24)

Acute perichondritis of the auricle is a bacterial infection of the perichondrium and underlying cartilage which usually develops following trauma to the skin of the pinna. A painful, red and swollen pinna following localized infection of the external ear, trauma or surgery, suggests the development of acute perichondritis.

Acute perichondritis occurs most commonly following lacerations or incisions which extend through the perichondrium. This type of acute

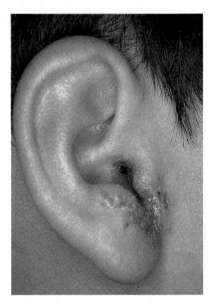

Fig. 6.23   Impetigo.

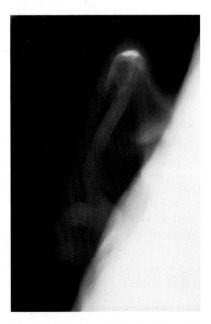

Fig. 6.22   Radiograph of the pinna of a patient who had severe frostbite many years before areas of calcification in the auricular cartilage appeared.

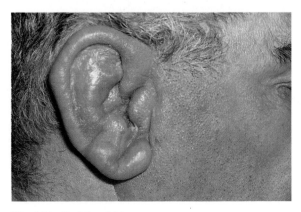

Fig. 6.24   Perichondritis.

bacterial infection is potentially serious because if untreated, the underlying auricular cartilage will become infected and ultimately necrotic with collapse of the pinna. Gram-negative bacteria, especially *Pseudomonas aeruginosa* and *Proteus*, are the usual causative organisms.

Treatment consists of an intravenous antibiotic which is effective against *Pseudomonas* (pending receipt of culture and sensitivity reports) combined with a broad-spectrum antibiotic, and the topical application of local compresses of Burrow's solution. If a subperichondrial abscess forms, then surgical incisions through the perichondrium with drainage of the infected material and the insertion of packing impregnated with an appropriate topical antibiotic will be required.

In severe cases the infection may spread to involve the outer part of the external auditory canal and radical surgery may be necessary.

Creased lobule (Fig. 6.25)

The appearance of a crease running across the skin of the lobule is a minor deformity which does not appear until later life. Most commonly the crease begins where the ear lobe attaches to the head and angles diagonally downwards and backwards to the edge of the lobule. This sign is associated with increasing age and also independently with increased incidence of obstructive coronary artery disease.

Bifid lobule (Fig. 6.26)

Congenital malformations or reduplications of the lobule are relatively rare. In the patient in Figure 6.26, there has been a failure in the fusion of the hillocks resulting in a bifid lobule. This is of no clinical significance. A similar appearance may result from careless ear piercing, or may be seen as a 'cut-out' deformity resulting from the forcible tearing of a pendular earring from the lobule (Fig. 6.27).

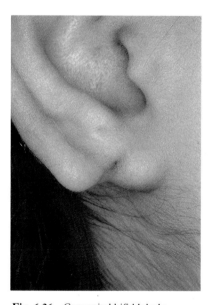

Fig. 6.26   Congenital bifid lobule.

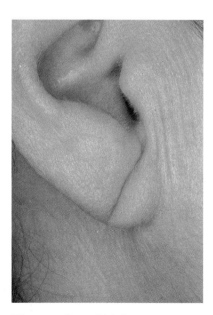

Fig. 6.25   Creased lobule.

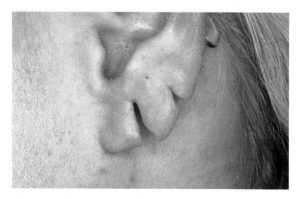

Fig. 6.27   Post-traumatic bifid lobule, resulting from the forcible tearing of an earring from the lobule.

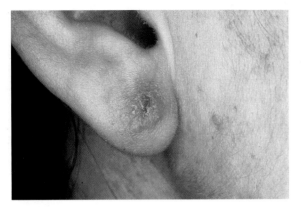

Fig. 6.28   Infected earring tract.

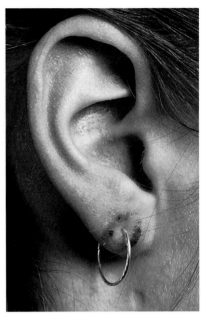

Fig. 6.29   Metal contact dermatitis of the lobule.

Infected earring tract (Fig. 6.28)

Localized infection within the epithelial-lined fistula tract of a pierced ear is usually the result of poor hygiene. On examination there will be localized tenderness, erythema, swelling and occasionally crusting. Pressure on the lobule will frequently expel a tiny drop of pus.

This type of infection can usually be avoided by good personal hygiene. If the infection does not respond to topical antibiotic therapy the earring may need to be removed.

Metal contact dermatitis of the lobule

A localized area of contact dermatitis (Fig. 6.29) is frequently seen under an earring. Cutaneous allergy (contact dermatitis) to base metals, especially to nickel, may develop when the gold plating covering a poor quality earring wears off and the underlying metal comes into direct contact with the underlying skin of the lobule. Concomitant infection may aggravate the inflammatory response and obliterate the earring tract.

Contact dermatitis

Contact dermatitis of the external ear is relatively common and can frequently be confused with infectious otitis externa. The offending allergen may be a topical medication such as neomycin, or one of the ingredients of topical ear drops, an ear mould, or an earring. One important differentiating feature is that patients with contact dermatitis complain primarily of itching rather than pain. Another important diagnostic clue is a track-like extension of the allergic inflammatory response below the ear as the discharge carries the allergen along.

The skin of the external ear may display a marked reaction to the allergen to which the patient has become sensitized. In the patient shown in Figure 6.30, the conchal bowl is red and swollen from a reaction to a topical ear preparation containing neomycin. Reactions may also occur to the materials used to make ear moulds (Fig. 6.31) or earrings (Fig. 6.29).

Treatment consists of avoiding the offending allergen and the topical application of a mild steroid-containing cream to the involved areas.

Hypertrophic scars and keloids

Keloids are the result of an abnormality in the wound healing process whereby excessive bulk is produced at the site of cutaneous injury, most commonly a laceration or a surgical incision, e.g. after ear piercing or surgical incisions around the ear. Keloids occur more commonly in blacks than in whites and develop most frequently in the second and third decades of life.

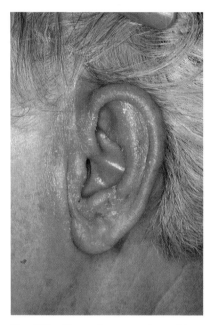

Fig. 6.30   Neomycin contact dermatitis.

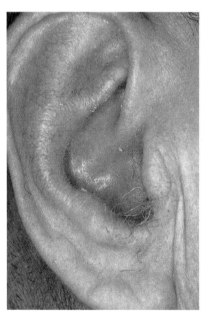

Fig. 6.31   Ear mould contact dermatitis (reaction to material used to make ear mould).

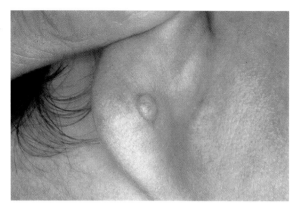

Fig. 6.32   Hypertrophic scar secondary to ear piercing.

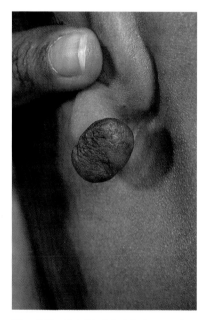

Fig. 6.33   Keloid of the lobule secondary to ear piercing.

A keloid should be differentiated from a simple hypertrophic scar. Hypertrophic scars (Fig. 6.32) remain within the confines of the wound and flatten spontaneously over 1 or more years. By contrast, keloids (Fig. 6.33) not only persist but extend beyond the site of the original injury.

While there is no uniformly effective treatment for an established keloid, they may be prevented by avoiding surgical incisions in susceptible individuals. If a keloid appears following cutaneous injury, the injection of a steroid into the base of the keloid is sometimes helpful. An unsightly keloid may be excised, and the margins of the excision site injected with steroids. Unfortunately there is a high incidence of recurrence. In the case shown in Figure 6.33, the keloid developed following ear piercing.

Post-traumatic epidermal inclusion cyst

Fragments of cutaneous epithelium may become trapped in the dermis of the lobule following ear piercing. If this happens, an epidermoid cyst (Fig. 6.34) will frequently develop from the entrapped remnants.

Epidermal cysts

Epidermal cysts are slow-growing, round, firm intradermal cysts that arise most commonly from the infundibula of the hair follicles. Clinically these cysts appear as smooth, round, doughy masses (Fig. 6.35), which may have a tiny surface

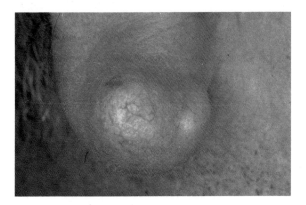

Fig. 6.34 Post-traumatic epidermoid cyst of the lobule secondary to ear piercing.

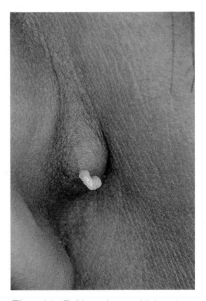

Fig. 6.35 Epidermal cyst with keratin debris being expressed.

opening. The overlying skin is frequently yellowish-white in colour due to the mass of pure white keratin contained within the cyst. Note the cheesy debris which is being expressed from the cyst in Figure 6.36.

The favoured sites for the development of epidermal cysts are along the post-auricular sulcus and the medial aspect of the lobule at its junction with the face.

If an epidermal cyst becomes infected, the lining of the cyst may rupture and the keratin squames within the cyst may spill out into the surrounding soft tissue. If this happens, an acute foreign body granulomatous reaction will develop in response to the keratin squames. Clinically, this may give rise to local tenderness. Epidermal cysts which are cosmetically displeasing or which have become repeatedly infected should be excised. If the cyst wall is incompletely removed, the cyst will probably recur.

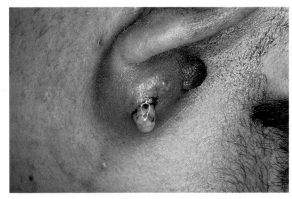

Fig. 6.36 Infected epidermal cyst just after incision.

Chronic infective dermatitis (eczema) (Fig. 6.37)

Healthy skin will usually provide an effective physical and chemical barrier against the numerous bacteria and fungi present in our environment. Under conditions of repeated trauma, moisture or maceration, the skin may lose this effective barrier. The result may be an acute or chronic superficial infection of the epidermis by bacteria, fungi, or a mixture of both organisms. Pruritis is the common feature in

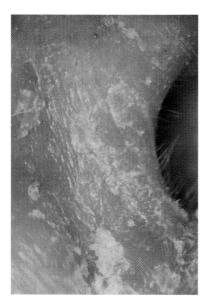

Fig. 6.37 Eczema.

chronic infective dermatitis and may provoke the patient into repeatedly scratching the involved area (neurodermatitis).

The infecting organisms may be either bacterial (most commonly *Staphylococcus aureus* or *Streptococcus*) or fungal (most commonly *Candida albicans*) or not infrequently a mixture of both. These superficial infections respond well to topical antibiotic or antifungal therapy combined with good hygiene. If the infection does not respond to the initial topical medication, a culture of the involved area should be taken for both bacteria and fungi and the medication adjusted accordingly. If the infection still does not respond, a biopsy may be needed to establish the diagnosis.

Psoriasis

The skin of the external ear can be affected by a host of dermatological disorders, including psoriasis (Fig. 6.38). Psoriasis vulgaris is a hereditary disorder of the skin which is characterized by an increased rate of epidermal cell replication. This chronic relapsing dermatosis is characterized by sharply defined, dry, erythematous patches covered with adherent, silvery-white scales. If the scales are removed by gentle scraping, fine punctate

bleeding points may be seen (the Auspitz sign).

When psoriasis involves the external ear, the patient may have typical lesions on the auricle (Fig. 6.38). Psoriasis may involve the external ear and the entrance to the external canal (Fig 6.39), but is rarely found in the deep meatus. The ear canal may be occluded by a toothpaste-like accumulation of keratin debris. If psoriasis is suspected in an otherwise asymptomatic patient, with persistent accumulation of debris in the canal, the elbows and the scalp should be inspected, as these are the most common sites for psoriasis.

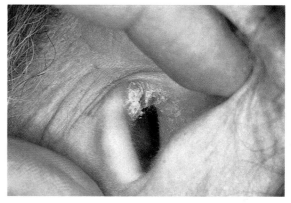

Fig. 6.38 Psoriasis.

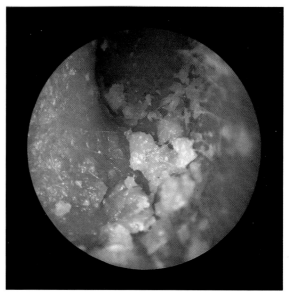

Fig. 6.39 Psoriasis affecting the skin of the cartilaginous external canal.

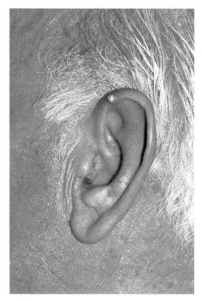

Fig. 6.40   Gouty tophus.

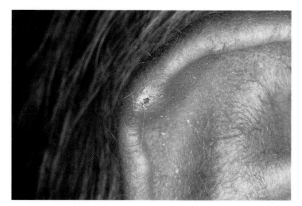

Fig. 6.41   Chondrodermatitis nodularis helicus chronica.

Gouty tophus

In advanced cases of gout, a deposit of urate crystals may appear on the helix as a tophus (Fig. 6.40); however, with modern medical treatment, this finding is now unusual. Gouty tophi present as painful skin-covered nodules which occur most commonly on the helix. On palpation the nodule is gritty, and yellow crystal-like structures may occasionally be seen through the skin.

Chondrodermatitis nodularis helicus chronica (Winkler's nodule)

Chondrodermatitis nodularis helicus chronica is the elaborate but descriptive name given to a discrete, firm, raised and frequently tender or even painful nodule which is usually located on the apex of the helix of the ear (Fig. 6.41). This lesion occurs primarily in middle-aged and elderly males, and is the result of solar damage to the skin covering the top of the pinna with resulting late solar elastosis. Repeated minor trauma and the poor blood supply to the helical rim are responsible for degeneration of the skin and the underlying dermis and auricular cartilage. A central epidermal channel

or pit (which develops for the purpose of transepidermal extrusion of the degenerated dermal collagen) is commonly seen. Treatment is excision of the nodule and the underlying degenerating cartilage.

Solar keratosis

Solar keratoses are considered to be premalignant lesions which arise on those areas of the skin which have been repeatedly exposed to the sun. These lesions occur most commonly in fair-skinned individuals after the third decade of life. Clinically, solar keratoses appear as dry, rough, adherent and scaly lesions (Fig. 6.42). Occasionally, solar keratoses produce a circum-scribed conical hyperkeratotic excrescence, which is termed a cutaneous horn (Fig. 6.43).

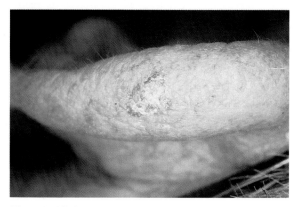

Fig. 6.42   Solar keratosis.

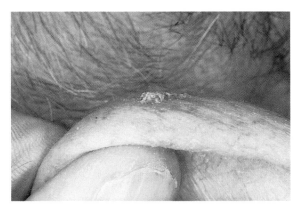

Fig. 6.43 Solar keratosis (cutaneous horn).

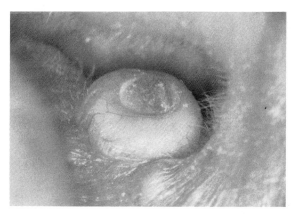

Fig. 6.45 Keratoacanthoma.

Although a solar keratosis may develop over time into a squamous cell carcinoma, the tumour that develops is usually less malignant than the usual squamous cell carcinoma which arises de novo. Because solar keratoses are pre-malignant they should be excised.

Pigmented lesions

Pigmented lesions (Fig. 6.44) frequently occur on the external ear. The presence of an enlarging or darkly pigmented lesion should, however, always arouse the examiner's suspicion to the possibility that this may in fact represent a malignant melanoma. This lesion was a pigmented naevus.

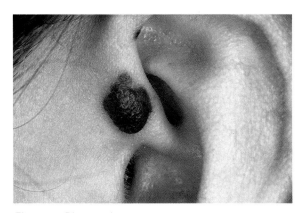

Fig. 6.44 Pigmented naevus.

Keratoacanthoma (Fig 6.45)

Keratoacanthomas are benign, usually solitary, rapidly developing epithelial neoplasms that arise most frequently on the sun-exposed areas of fair-skinned elderly individuals. The lesion consists of a firm, dome-shaped nodule which has skin-coloured rolled edges and a central crater (Fig. 6.45) filled with keratin debris. Keratoacanthomas usually begin as an erythematous papule that enlarges rapidly over 2–8 weeks to reach a maximum size of 1–2 cm; if left alone it will involute spontaneously within 6–12 months, leaving behind a puckered and often unsightly scar.

Unfortunately, keratoacanthomas resemble squamous cell carcinomas both clinically and histologically. When the diagnosis is in doubt, and to avoid the scarring that accompanies spontaneous involution, an excisional biopsy is usually indicated.

Basal cell carcinoma

The presence of persistent ulceration of the external ear should suggest the possibility of an underlying malignancy (Fig. 6.46). This patient had been treated for many months for a chronic infection of the external ear when, in fact, she had an extensive basal cell carcinoma involving the conchal bowl. The diagnosis was established by biopsy and the tumour responded to radiotherapy.

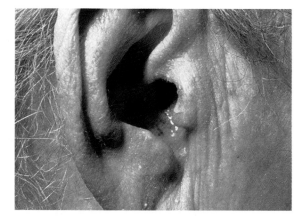

Fig. 6.46   Basal cell carcinoma.

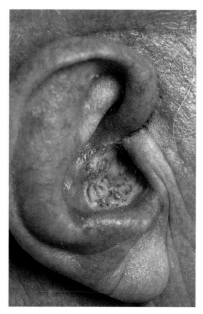

Fig. 6.48   Squamous cell carcinoma.

Squamous cell carcinoma (Fig. 6.48)

Squamous cell carcinoma of the auricle is a relatively uncommon malignant tumour which usually arises from keratinocytes which have been damaged by an exogenous agent such as sunlight, X-rays or radium burns. The malignancy occurs frequently in persons of fair complexion who have experienced long exposure to sunlight.

Clinically, a squamous cell carcinoma may appear as an indurated papule, plaque or nodule which is frequently eroded, crusted and ulcerated. Rapid growth in the size of the lesion, tenderness to palpation, crusting and ulceration are all signs that should alert the physician to presence of squamous cell carcinoma. On palpation the lesion is hard and may be fixed to the underlying structures. In rare instances there may be spread to the regional lymph nodes.

Treatment requires an excisional biopsy combined with resection of any involved lymph nodes and in some cases postoperative radiotherapy.

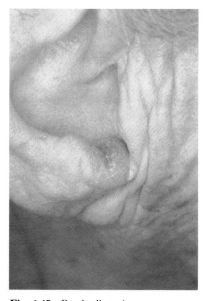

Fig. 6.47   Basal cell carcinoma.

More commonly, the proliferation of basal cells creates a raised indurated nodule with firm pearly edges (Fig. 6.47). A small central crust is frequently present, underneath which is a central ulcer.

Post-auricular scar

This post-auricular scar (Fig. 6.49) indicates that the patient has almost certainly had previous tympanomastoid surgery.

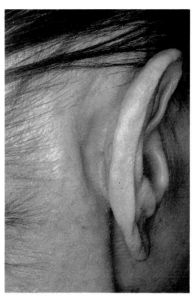

Fig. 6.50   Depressed post-auricular scar.

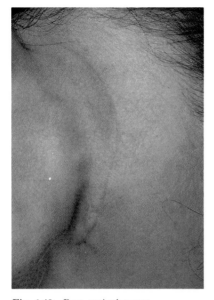

Fig. 6.49   Post-auricular scar.

Depressed post-auricular scar

The post-auricular sulcus of this patient (Fig. 6.50) shows not only a post-auricular scar but also significant depression over the mastoid process caused by removal of the mastoid cortex and a failure to effect proper closure of the fascial layer.

Mastoid fistula (Fig. 6.51)

It is important always to look behind the pinna, since significant pathology (e.g. basal cell or squamous cell carcinoma) in this area may otherwise be easily overlooked. This patient has a fistulous communication between the post-auricular skin and the mastoid antrum.

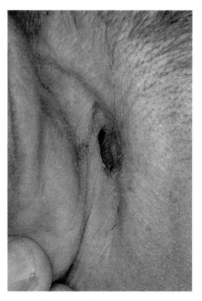

Fig. 6.51   Mastoid fistula.

7. Diseases of the external auditory canal

HAEMATOMA OF THE EXTERNAL CANAL

Definition
A haematoma is a subepidermal collection of blood.

Aetiology
Haematomas of the skin of the external auditory canal are usually the result of direct physical trauma to the thin and delicate skin of the deep external canal from an object which has been inserted into the ear canal, e.g. matchstick, cotton-tipped applicator etc.

Symptoms
Haematomas are usually asymptomatic and indicate only that the skin of the ear canal has recently been traumatized.

Clinical appearances
The haematoma will appear initially as a bright red linear streak along the skin of the canal (Fig. 7.1). Larger haematomas may raise the skin of the canal, appearing as a red bleb (Fig. 7.2). Over time, the bright red colour will darken and the subepidermal collection of blood will be slowly resorbed.

Treatment guidelines
Haematomas require no treatment.

LACERATIONS OF THE EXTERNAL CANAL

Definition
A tear of the skin lining the external auditory canal.

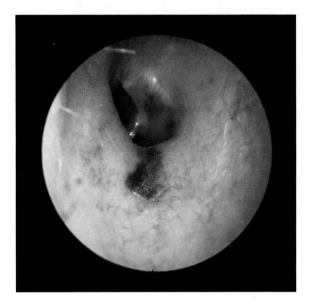

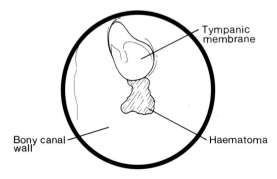

Fig. 7.1 Traumatic haematoma. Note the small linear haematoma on the floor of the bony canal. This type of haematoma is frequently an incidental finding in those patients who regularly clean their ears.

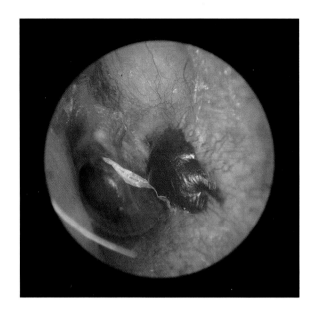

Symptoms

The principal symptoms are bleeding and pain, but hearing loss can occur if the meatus fills with blood.

Otoscopic appearances

In most cases a small tear in the superficial canal skin will be seen and occasionally a flap of skin may have been raised (Fig. 7.3). There may be evidence of haematoma (Figs 7.1 and 7.2), recent bleeding (Fig. 7.4), blood clot (Fig. 7.5) or crust which may have accumulated within the meatus. The ear should be carefully examined to ensure that the laceration is confined to the external canal skin and does not involve the tympanic membrane or middle ear.

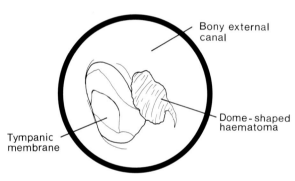

Fig. 7.2 Traumatic haematoma. There is a large dome-shaped haematoma in the skin of the posterior bony canal.

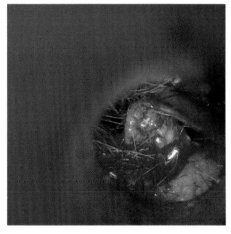

Fig. 7.3 Traumatic laceration. A flap of skin has been raised from the floor of the cartilaginous canal.

Aetiology

While the skin of the deep meatus is extremely thin and easily traumatized it is well protected from external trauma and it is usually the skin of the more accessible superficial meatus which is the site of lacerations. These lacerations occur most frequently as the result of inadvertent self-manipulation by the patient. A fingernail, hairpin, matchstick or cotton-tipped applicator is often the direct cause of the injury. Less commonly, lacerations may result from the clumsy insertion of a speculum, ear syringe or wax hook into the canal. They may also result from unskilled attempts at foreign body removal.

Treatment guidelines

The bleeding from a laceration is generally self-limiting and the ear should simply be kept dry to avoid possible infection. In those cases in which the laceration may have been contaminated, the use of a suitable topical antibiotic ear drop is recommended. Any clot in the meatus should be carefully removed so that the deeper structures can be examined. It is also much easier to remove a fresh, soft, jelly-like clot before it turns into a stony, hard, black, tar-like mass (Fig. 7.5).

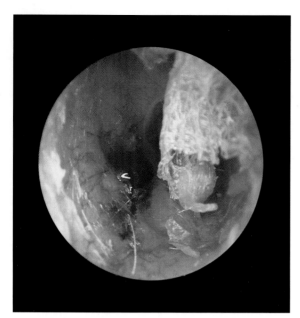

Fig. 7.4   Traumatic laceration. Note the droplet of fresh blood which is oozing from a small laceration in the floor of the bony canal. If the bleeding is not stopped, the canal may fill with blood.

Most lacerations of the external ear canal heal completely without visible scarring. In a few cases a keratin foreign body granuloma develops, due to the implantation of keratin squames into the dermis. In these cases exuberant granulation tissue forms, usually within 1–2 weeks after the injury. Removal of the granulation tissue and the implanted foreign material (superficial corneocytes) is usually required to allow healing.

A small epithelial inclusion cyst will occasionally develop if epithelial cells have been trapped in the dermis (Fig. 7.6). These tiny cysts appear as a pearly-white, round swelling in the skin of the external canal and rarely enlarge.

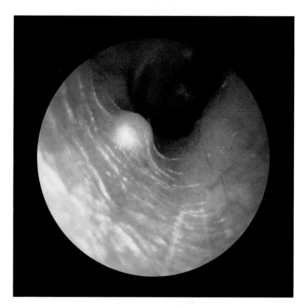

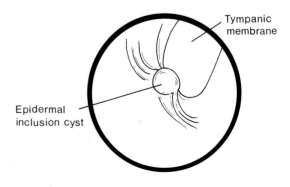

Fig. 7.5   Old blood clot. The external auditory canal is totally blocked by a stony, hard, tar-like plug of desiccated clot.

Fig. 7.6   Epidermal inclusion cyst. A small pearly-white epidermal inclusion cyst is seen on the posteroinferior canal wall.

KERATOSIS OBTURANS

Definition

Blockage of the deep meatus by a hard plug of white keratin debris (Fig. 7.7).

Aetiology

The normal self-cleansing mechanism of the external ear canal is the net result of the finely co-ordinated processes of keratin maturation and lateral cell migration. In keratosis obturans, these mechanisms are non-functional. While the aetiology of keratosis obturans remains unclear, it appears that there is an increased rate of desquamation of corneocytes within the deep canal and a failure of the normal outward migration of these epithelial cells from the surface of the tympanic membrane laterally along the surface of the skin lining the external canal. The result is an accumulation of keratin within the meatus.

This plug of accumulated keratin (Fig. 7.8) remains stuck within the deep canal, exerting pressure on the walls and gradually stimulating resorption of the bony walls of the surrounding canal, which is clinically seen as widening (Fig. 7.9). Increased hyperaemia of the external canal also seems to play a significant role.

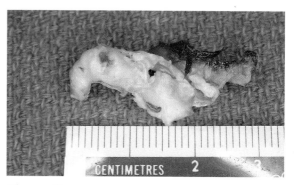

Fig. 7.8 Keratosis obturans. The large white plug of compressed keratin seen in Figure 7.7 has been removed using instruments under the operating microscope.

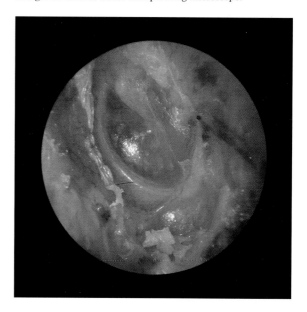

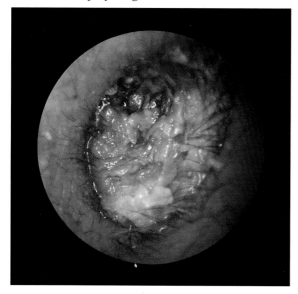

Fig. 7.7 Keratosis obturans. A large plug of keratin debris is occluding the external meatus and is adherent to the skin of the canal.

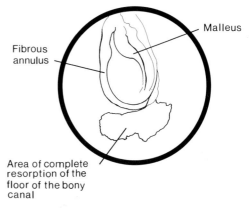

Fig. 7.9 Keratosis obturans. Over time, the slowly enlarging keratin plug has caused resorption of the inferior deep bony canal wall. The fibrous annulus appears to be hanging in mid-air.

Symptoms

A conductive hearing loss is the most common symptom. Severe pain may result from laceration of the canal skin during an attempt at cleansing with the development of an otitis externa or a keratin foreign body granuloma. In some cases keratosis obturans is associated with bronchiectasis and chronic sinusitis.

Otoscopic appearances

The bony meatus is occluded by a plug of compressed pearly-white keratin debris (Fig. 7.7). On palpation this plug is found to be very hard. After removal of this plug of compressed keratin squames, hyperaemia of the underlying canal skin and superficial granulations arising from the underlying inflamed skin are frequently seen. In long-standing cases, a generalized widening of the deep bony canal may occur as a result of the slow expansion of the keratin plug (Fig. 7.9). In rare cases, the bony erosion caused by the gradually enlarging keratin plug may be so extensive that an automastoidectomy is carried out (Fig. 7.10). In any event, great care must be taken in removing the plug because the erosion may uncap the facial nerve in its vertical portion and also expose the jugular bulb.

Treatment guidelines

The aim of treatment is firstly to remove the keratin plug safely and completely, and secondly to prevent any recurrence. The hardness of the keratin plug and its adherence to the underlying skin may make the removal of the plug technically difficult, requiring the use of the operating microscope, and in some cases a general anaesthetic may be necessary. Any inflammation of the ear canal skin or secondary otitis externa should be treated with a suitable topical antibiotic ear drop. As this idiopathic condition has a tendency to recur, these patients should be seen in follow-up on a regular basis, so that any accumulation of keratin can be readily removed before the lumen of the canal becomes totally obstructed.

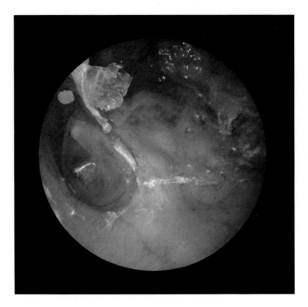

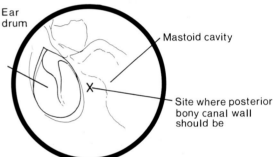

Fig. 7.10. Automastoidectomy resulting from long-neglected keratosis obturans. In this patient the pressure from the slowly enlarging plug of compressed keratin squames has caused resorption of the entire posterior wall of the bony external ear canal and a large portion of the mastoid, resulting in an automastoidectomy.

BENIGN OSTEITIS OF THE EXTERNAL EAR CANAL (SYNONYM: CHOLESTEATOMA OF THE EXTERNAL AUDITORY CANAL)

Definition

This distinct clinical entity is characterized by a localized ulceration in the skin of the floor of the bony external auditory canal with osteitis and sequestration of the underlying exposed tympanic bone.

Aetiology

Although the precise aetiology is unclear, benign osteitis of the tympanic bone appears to result from a traumatic laceration and subsequent ulceration of the skin of the deep meatus. This ulceration, if combined with infection, results in necrosis of the underlying periosteum with exposure, infection (osteitis) and ultimately sequestration of the underlying tympanic bone. Patients with benign osteitis of the tympanic bone are usually elderly and frequently suffer from chronic lung disease.

Symptoms

While the symptoms are minor and variable, the most common symptom is a persistent dull otalgia with or without otorrhoea. Most cases are unilateral, although benign osteitis ·may occur bilaterally. Hearing loss (with the exception of presbycusis which is not infrequently encountered in this age group) is not a feature of this disease unless there has been a secondary accumulation of debris within the ear canal.

Otoscopic appearances

The typical ulceration in the skin covering the floor of the deep meatus may not be seen until the ear canal has been cleaned and the area debrided. The entire ulcerated area may be covered with a smooth yellowish layer of inspissated serum-like exudate which can on first glance resemble cerumen or even normal deep canal skin.

In some patients, fresh granulations and an accumulation of white keratin debris may be found covering the base of the ulcer (Fig. 7.11). Following cleansing and debridement of the base of the ulcer, exposed abnormally yellowish tympanic bone will always be found (Fig. 7.12).

Treatment guidelines

The most appropriate method of treatment depends on the severity of the symptoms, the

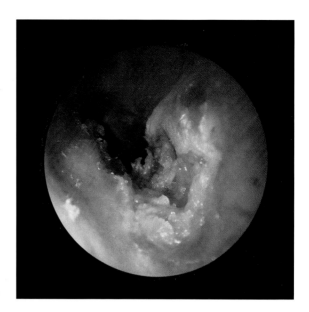

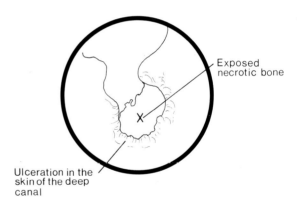

Exposed necrotic bone

Ulceration in the skin of the deep canal

Fig. 7.11 Benign osteitis of the tympanic bone. Note the ulceration in the skin of the floor of the bony canal. The margins of the ulcer are hyperkeratotic.

extent of the osteitis and the general health of the often elderly and debilitated patient. In most cases, the clinical course of this disease is relatively mild. Simple transcanal curettage with removal of the sequestrum and granulation tissue with exposure of healthy bone will usually allow epithelialization of the cutaneous ulceration and resolution.

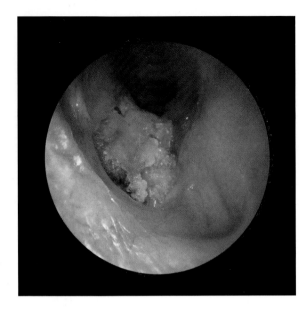

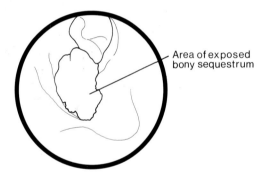

Area of exposed
bony sequestrum

Fig. 7.12   Benign osteitis of the tympanic bone. Note the yellowish exposed sequestrating bone which can be seen in the floor of the deep canal.

FOREIGN BODIES

Definition

Any foreign material located within the external auditory canal.

Aetiology

A wide selection of foreign bodies have been discovered in the external auditory canal. In children, small plastic beads, toy building materials, foam rubber and paper are currently in vogue, whilst in adults a forgotten piece of cotton wool is commonly encountered by the examiner.

Symptoms

Pain, irritation, hearing loss and otorrhoea can all occur. Relatively inert materials may produce no symptoms whatsoever and may only be discovered inadvertently during a routine otoscopic examination whereas vegetable material tends to cause a localized external otitis. Occasionally, the fluttering or scratching movements of a living insect in the external canal will cause considerable distress.

Otoscopic appearances

The type of foreign body present can usually be recognized without difficulty (Figs 7.13–7.15), unless wax or secondary infection with discharge obscures the picture.

Treatment guidelines

The aim is to remove the foreign body as safely and expeditiously as possible, while avoiding damage to the delicate skin of the external auditory canal, the tympanic membrane and the

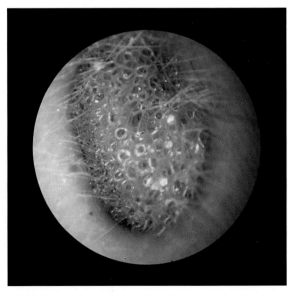

Fig. 7.13   Foreign body. A piece of blue sponge rubber is seen blocking the external auditory canal.

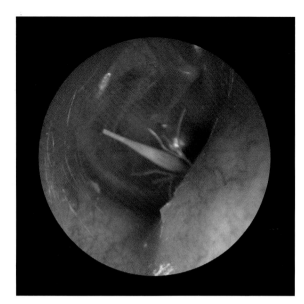

Fig. 7.14 Foreign body. A small seed can be seen lying against the tympanic membrane. This type of foreign body can be easily removed by syringing.

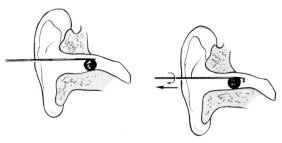

Fig. 7.16 Technique of wax removal. The use of a blunt wax hook for the removal of a foreign body. A blunt right-angle probe is inserted into the external canal and past the foreign body without touching either the canal wall or the foreign body. After insertion, the probe is rotated and the foreign body gently rolled out of the canal.

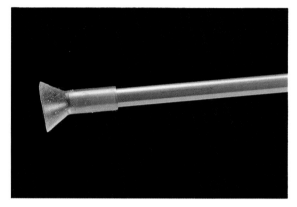

Fig. 7.17 The Schuknecht foreign body remover.

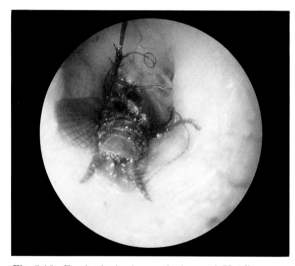

Fig. 7.15 Foreign body. A recently deceased *Blatella germanicus* can be seen lying on its back in the deep canal.

ossicles. The method of choice depends on the type of foreign body present. Smooth, hard, round objects such as beads are best removed with a blunt wax hook (Fig. 7.16), while aural crocodile forceps are more suitable for those foreign bodies which present an edge and can be easily grasped, e.g. paper, foam rubber or cotton wool.

A small aural suction tube of the Bellucci pattern is invaluable in many cases. Dr Harold Schuknecht of Harvard, USA has invented a special funnel-shaped suction tip foreign body remover (Fig. 7.17) which can be used for the removal of round foreign bodies.

If the foreign material is fragmented and not totally blocking the canal an aural syringe can be used to flush it out. Insects are best floated out by filling the canal with water or oil. This is a simple measure which may prevent a camping holiday from being spoilt.

In unco-operative patients, and especially in children, it may be impossible to remove the foreign body safely and painlessly. A short general anaesthetic is then advisable to avoid the possibility of damaging the external canal and tympanic membrane.

EXOSTOSES

Definition

An exostosis is a benign, slowly growing, dome-shaped area of localized bony hypertrophy arising from the medial surface of the tympanic bone (the bone of the deep external ear canal).

Aetiology

Exostoses appear to arise in susceptible individuals in response to the repeated stimulation of the bony external canal by cold water. The initial cold-induced vasoconstriction of the deep canal is followed by a reactive hyperaemia and a stimulation of the periosteum lining the medial surface of the tympanic bone which lays down consecutive layers of subperiosteal bone. A history of frequent aquatic activities (swimming, diving, surfing etc.) will often be obtained in these patients. Exostoses are usually multiple, occur bilaterally and are more common in males than females.

Symptoms

Exostoses are usually asymptomatic unless they become large enough to cause a hearing loss by blocking the external canal or entrapping wax.

Otoscopic appearances

Exostoses may be circumscribed (Fig. 7.18), or diffuse (Figs 7.19 and 7.20). They appear as small, hard, shiny, discrete round or oval excrescences, which are sometimes pedunculated and may be single or multiple. The skin overlying the exostosis is usually thinner and paler than normal. A single exostosis can be differentiated from a foreign body or cyst by gentle palpation with a blunt, ring-ended probe. In advanced cases three large exostoses arising from opposing sides of the canal can reduce the lumen to a tri-radiate star—the 'Mercedes Benz' sign.

Further investigations

When multiple exostoses prevent the examiner from seeing the tympanic membrane, audio-

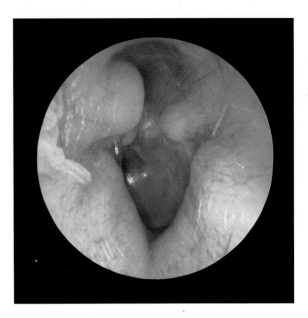

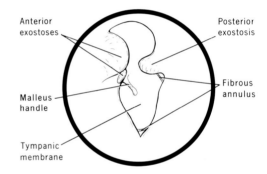

Fig. 7.18   Exostoses. Two exostoses are present—a large sessile anterior exostosis and a smaller pedunculated posterior exostosis. The tympanic membrane, malleus handle and fibrous annulus are visible behind the exostoses.

metric tests and tympanometry may be useful in assessing middle ear function.

Treatment guidelines

If the entry of cold water into the ear canal is prevented by wearing suitable earplugs, then the exostoses will not continue to enlarge. Since most exostoses are asymptomatic, they usually require

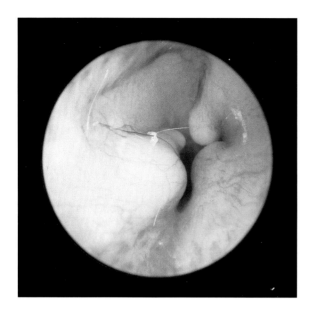

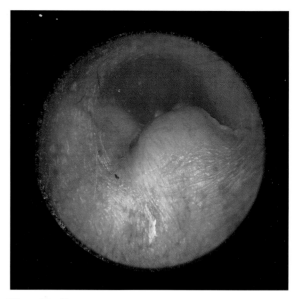

Fig. 7.20 Exostoses. Multiple exostoses are blocking the lumen of the bony external canal.

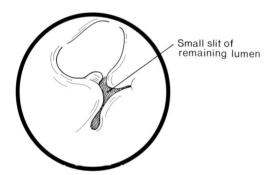

Small slit of remaining lumen

Fig. 7.19 Exostoses. Multiple coalescent exostoses are blocking the lumen of this patient's bony external auditory canal. A small narrowed lumen can be seen in the anteroinferior quadrant.

OSTEOMAS (Fig. 7.21)

Definition

Osteomas of the external auditory canal are benign bony tumours arising from the tympanic bone.

Aetiology

The aetiology of osteomas is unknown. They are considered to be a true benign bony tumour and, unlike exostoses, osteomas do not develop as a reactive phenomenon.

Symptoms

Unlike exostoses, osteomas usually trap wax and keratin debris in the deep meatus, thereby producing a conductive hearing loss.

Otoscopic appearances

Unlike exostoses, osteomas are usually solitary, appearing as a bony hard sessile mass covered by normal deep canal skin (Fig. 7.21). The 'bony' nature of these tumours can readily be determined by palpation.

no treatment. In cases where entrapment of wax occurs or chronic otitis externa develops, repeated debridement with the operating microscope may be required on a regular basis. In those rare instances when the exostoses totally occlude the external canal (Fig. 7.20) or prevent a permeatal approach to the middle ear, a transcanal surgical removal is then indicated.

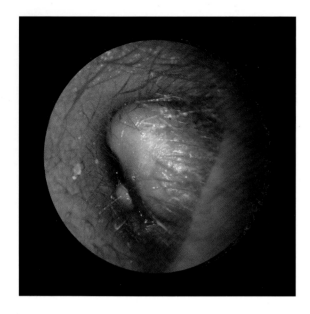

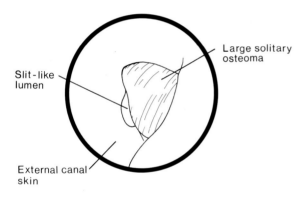

Large solitary osteoma

Slit-like lumen

External canal skin

Fig. 7.21   Osteoma. Note the large solitary osteoma which is extending out into the lumen of the cartilaginous canal.

Treatment guidelines

If an osteoma becomes symptomatic by occluding the lumen of the canal or by trapping wax and keratin debris within the canal, it should be removed.

ACUTE CIRCUMSCRIBED OTITIS EXTERNA (FURUNCLE)

Definition

A staphylococcal abscess arising from the base of a hair follicle, commonly referred to as a boil.

Furuncles can only occur in the outer cartilaginous part of the ear canal, since the skin of the inner two-thirds of the canal is hairless.

Aetiology

Furuncles usually result from the entry of pyogenic staphylococci into the skin of the canal.

Symptoms

Since the skin of the external canal is adherent to the underlying perichondrium, even a small furuncle will produce severe local pain, aggravated by movement of the pinna, pressure on the tragus or even chewing. Hearing loss is unusual but may be present if the external canal is occluded either by a large solitary furuncle or by oedema.

Otoscopic appearances

An extremely tender erythematous (red) localized swelling located in the outer hair-bearing portion of the external canal is typically seen (Fig. 7.22). It should be noted that a small furuncle may be missed on otoscopic examination if the aural speculum is inserted too deeply: when examining the ear, care must be taken always to examine the superficial part of the canal. The tympanic membrane is not involved in this condition; however, if the tympanic membrane cannot be inspected, either because it is obscured by a large furuncle or if the patient experiences such pain on examination that the speculum cannot be advanced into the deep meatus, the examiner must then consider all other causes of acute inflammatory ear disease, such as otitis media or mastoiditis. Enlargement of the lymph nodes between the mandible and the mastoid and pain on moving the tragus are common in furunculosis but are extremely unusual in middle ear infections.

Further investigations

A swab should be taken for culture and sensitivity of any purulent material present. In cases of recurrent furunculosis, further investigations to exclude an underlying systemic disease such as diabetes or a blood dyscrasia

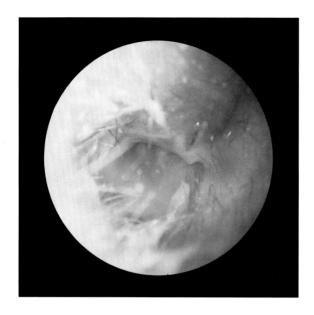

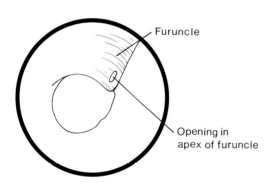

Fig. 7.22 Furuncle. A large, painful, pointing furuncle is visible on the posteroinferior canal wall.

should be considered. If there is doubt about the differentiation between mastoiditis and acute circumscribed otitis externa, mastoid X-rays should be obtained. In acute mastoiditis, X-rays will typically show clouding and coalescence of the mastoid air cells.

Treatment guidelines

If the furuncle is obviously pointing, it can be punctured with a large sterile hypodermic needle, bringing relief from pain. More commonly, however, the patient is seen at an early stage, when incision is of little value. A

wick of half-inch (1 cm) ribbon gauze—the best wick available today is the Pope Otowick, a small dried plug of compressed Merocel which can be easily inserted into the narrowed canal and which gradually expands once moistened—soaked in a solution of aluminium acetate (13%), or a mixture of acetic acid (2%) and propylene glycol diacetate (3%) can usually be gently inserted into the canal. These compounds are hygroscopic and produce relief of pain by reducing the swelling and stabilizing the canal during jaw movements. Analgesics and a full course of an oral broad-spectrum antibiotic are indicated. Penicillin is usually the drug of choice, but amoxycillin and potassium clavulanate acid will be preferred if the causative organism is suspected to be a penicillinase-producing strain.

ACUTE DIFFUSE OTITIS EXTERNA (SWIMMER'S EAR)

Definition

An acute, diffuse and painful bacterial infection of the skin of the external auditory canal.

Aetiology

The chief agents responsible for the development of acute diffuse otitis externa are local trauma and moisture. The patient may only reluctantly admit to the use of a fingernail, hair-grip (bobby pin) or cotton-tipped applicator to clean the ear. The entry of water after showering or swimming, or exposure to a hot and humid climate are also important predisposing factors. Gram-negative bacteria, principally *Pseudomonas aeruginosa*, can be cultured in almost every case.

Symptoms

These include pain, which is often severe, irritation, a blocked feeling within the ear, otorrhoea, itching and hearing loss when the canal is occluded by debris or swelling of the lining epithelium.

Otoscopic appearances

The skin of the external canal is swollen, extremely tender, and shiny in appearance (Fig.

7.23). A *peau d'orange* appearance is occasionally seen, due to lymphoedema. It is frequently impossible to examine the tympanic membrane if the lumen of the meatus is obliterated (Fig. 7.24).

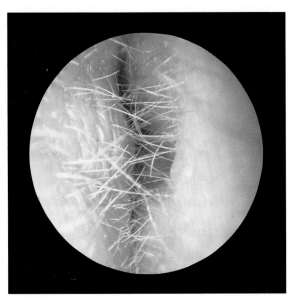

Fig. 7.23   Acute otitis externa. The cartilaginous external auditory canal is oedematous and the lumen is narrowed to a slit.

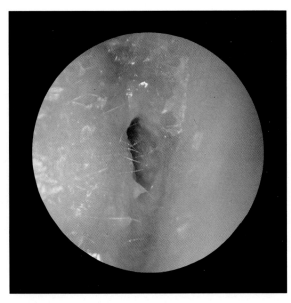

Fig. 7.24   Acute otitis externa. Note the swollen canal walls and the yellowish mucopurulent exudate.

In severe cases, the ear is so tender that even the gentlest movement of the pinna causes pain, and the introduction of the smallest speculum available is resisted by the patient. Whitish mucopurulent material is often present within the canal and usually wax is absent.

Treatment guidelines

If local treatment is to be effective, the canal must be thoroughly cleaned after taking a swab for bacterial and fungal cultures. In early cases, gentle cleaning of the canal with a cotton-tipped Jobson Horne probe will be effective. It is pointless to instil ear drops into a canal filled with debris since, in order for topical therapy to be effective, the medication must be able to make direct contact with the underlying skin of the canal.

If the lumen of the canal has been narrowed by oedematous skin, suction debridement under the microscope is preferred. In these cases, the patient will be unable to instil a topical preparation into the occluded ear canal and a Pope Otowick (Fig. 7.25) is gently eased as far as possible into the canal, moistened and then impregnated with a suitable topical antibiotic and anti-inflammatory preparation. This wick should be replaced on a daily basis until the swelling has subsided and the drops can be directly instilled into the canal. In severe cases the oral administration of non-steroidal anti-inflammatory preparations such as indomethacin may be of substantial value.

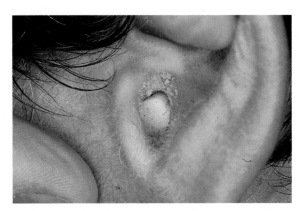

Fig. 7.25   Gauze wick. A selvedged ribbon gauze wick has been inserted into the patient's external auditory canal. The wick will help carry topical medication into the canal.

The most commonly prescribed topical ear drops contain an antibiotic effective against *Pseudomonas*, e.g. an aminoglycoside, together with a corticosteroid to reduce inflammation. The inclusion of a local anaesthetic in some preparations used for the treatment of acute diffuse otitis externa is probably not warranted, since reactive allergic dermatitis is a possibility, and if analgesia is required then systemic medication is preferred.

In chronic cases, resistant to therapy, care should be taken that one is not dealing with an aminoglycoside or other antibiotic skin sensitivity. This is an unusual but not unknown response to neomycin, which is a frequent ingredient in many antibiotic-containing ear drops. There may also be a sensitivity to other constituents of the topical preparation, including the carrier medium, such as propylene glycol.

If mucus is seen in the canal, then there is a high likelihood of a perforation in the tympanic membrane, since there are no mucus-producing glands within the external canal. Chronic cases of otitis externa may sometimes be caused by an unsuspected middle ear infection pouring secretions into the canal through a small perforation which cannot be seen because of the generalized swelling of the canal skin.

OTOMYCOSIS

Definition

A superficial fungal infection of the ear; usually located in the external auditory canal, it can also be found in the middle ear or in a mastoidectomy or fenestration cavity. Deep fungal infections involving the ear are extremely uncommon.

Aetiology

Candida albicans, Aspergillus niger, A. flavus and *A. fumigatus* are the organisms most commonly encountered. Predisposing factors include moisture, e.g. swimming or showering, and the previous use of topical antibiotic ear drops, especially those containing neomycin.

Symptoms

The symptoms of the otomycosis are itching, local irritation, persistent otorrhoea and pain. At an early stage the pain is often more severe than the clinical appearance would warrant, suggesting to the examiner the possibility of a mycotic infection.

Otoscopic appearances

In the early stages, examination generally reveals a cottonwool-like appearance or debris which resembles moist paper tissue. In advanced cases the ear canal may be filled with a whitish or creamy, thick material. There may be a fluffy appearance, due to the presence of tiny mycelia (Fig. 7.26). When the infection is caused by *A. niger*, it may be possible to identify the tiny greyish-black conidiophores or fruiting heads (Fig. 7.27). The underlying canal skin is often inflamed and granular, due to invasion by fungal mycelia (Fig. 7.28).

Further investigations

In many patients, the typical appearance of otomycosis is masked by debris and the correct

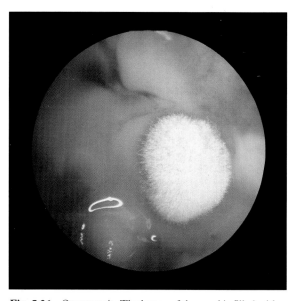

Fig. 7.26 Otomycosis. The lumen of the canal is filled with a creamy white mucopurulent exudate. Note the fluffy white diagnostic island which consists of the fungal hyphae of *Aspergillus* species.

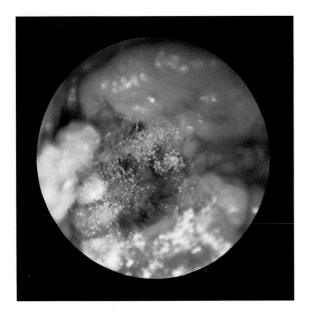

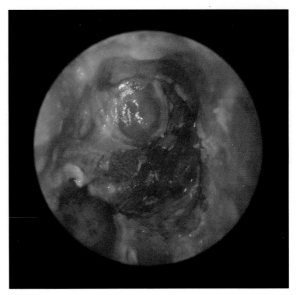

Fig. 7.28 Otomycosis: *Aspergillus niger*. This is the same ear as shown in Figure 7.26 after debridement. Note the ulceration of the skin of the deep canal and the granular tympanic membrane, due to invasion by *Aspergillus niger*.

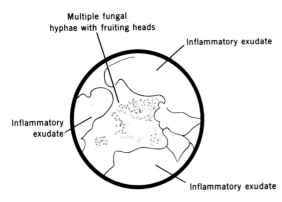

Multiple fungal
hyphae with fruiting heads

Inflammatory exudate

Inflammatory
exudate

Inflammatory exudate

Fig. 7.27 Otomycosis: *Aspergillus niger*. Numerous mycelia with brown fruiting heads are visible. A brownish-yellow mucopurulent exudate is present behind.

diagnosis can only be reached by specifically culturing a sample of the exudate for fungi. This is especially true for *Candida albicans* which has no specific visual diagnostic features. A swab should therefore be sent for both fungal and bacterial cultures in all cases of chronic otorrhoea. In most laboratories, fungal cultures on Saboraud's medium are not routinely performed and *must be specifically requested*.

Treatment guidelines

Thorough aural toilet by suction or dry-mopping with a cotton-tipped applicator to remove every vestige of debris is once again the cornerstone of effective treatment. Mastoid and fenestration cavities must be completely emptied of wax and infected material. An appropriate topical antifungal preparation is then applied. Refractory cases will require repeated aural toilet, with re-application of an antifungal agent, selected in the light of laboratory culture studies, several times a week to effect a cure.

In those cases of otomycosis caused by *Candida* species, nystatin ointment or lotion is usually effective, while in those cases caused by *Aspergillus* species, a 1% clotrimazole suspension is usually more effective.

The most effective method of treating both *Candida* and *Aspergillus* species is a single-dose coating of the external canal with pure clotrimazole powder following debridement.

CHRONIC OTITIS EXTERNA

Definition

A prolonged or recurrent diffuse inflammatory condition of the skin of the external auditory canal.

Aetiology

Acute diffuse otitis externa can become chronic if incompletely treated or if the initial predisposing factors (e.g. local trauma, moisture, etc.) remain. Many cases of chronic otitis externa are self-inflicted due to repeated contamination of the ear with water or by self-manipulation.

Chronic diffuse otitis externa can also occur secondarily to active chronic otitis media. The presence of pus in the ear canal arising from infected middle ear mucosa does not normally by itself induce infection of the canal skin, and it is probable that skin involvement develops only after scratching or inept aural toilet.

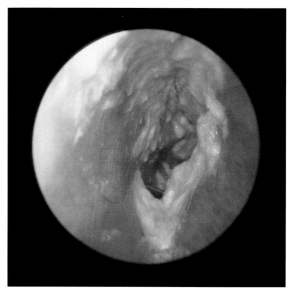

Fig. 7.29 Chronic otitis externa. The skin of the external bony canal is thickened and the lumen is blocked with a yellowish-brown plug of infected cerumen.

Symptoms

The symptoms of chronic otitis externa consist primarily of itching, fullness, hearing loss and otorrhoea, whilst severe pain is not generally a prominent feature. Normal desquamation and ventilation of the ear canal are impaired and since the ear tends to itch and feel blocked, a vicious cycle of itching and scratching is established.

Otoscopic appearances

The otoscopic appearances in chronic otitis externa can be quite variable. The skin of the meatus is often thickened, with partial or complete stenosis sometimes occurring. Foul-smelling debris is usually found within the meatus (Figs 7.29 and 7.30), although in some patients the only signs of chronic otitis externa may be a slight redness of the epithelium and a complete absence of any wax or debris.

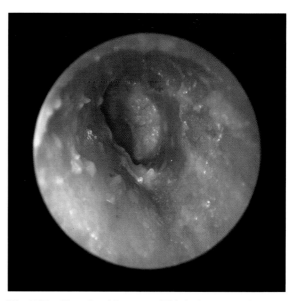

Fig. 7.30 Chronic otitis externa. This is the same patient as shown in Figure 7.29 after the plug of material has been debrided from the external canal. Notice the narrowed lumen caused by chronic thickening and fibrosis within the lining skin. A small haematoma which occurred during cleaning is seen on the anterior canal wall.

Further investigations

The first step is to send a swab for bacterial and fungal studies to identify the causative organisms and to assist in the selection of an appropriate topical antibiotic or antimycotic agent. The possibility of an underlying dermatological disorder, systemic disease, or even a malignancy should always be considered in unresponsive cases.

Treatment guidelines

The aim of treatment is to restore the skin of the meatus to its normal state. In practice this can be extremely difficult; despite energetic prolonged therapy, many of these patients are only free of disease for short periods of time.

The mainstay of treatment is thorough aural toilet and a modification of any factors in the patient's behaviour which have contributed to the development of the disease, e.g. scratching and exposure of the ear to moisture. Thorough aural toilet can be accomplished either by dry-mopping with cotton wool or by suction under microscopic control. It is crucial to remove every vestige of debris from the ear canal if topical therapy is to be successful.

In those cases in which the lumen is moderately narrow, a selvedged half-inch (1 cm) ribbon gauze wick saturated with Burrows solution is then introduced into the canal. If the canal is almost obliterated and will not admit a wick, triamcinolone otic ointment can usually be inserted into the ear canal from a syringe fitted with a soft fine polyethylene tip. Repeated thorough toilet with the reapplication of topical therapy modified in the light of results obtained from culture studies is generally rewarded by improvement. Here again, the examiner should be on the look-out for allergic reactions to the medications used, or the presence of a more serious underlying disease.

ACQUIRED EXTERNAL CANAL STENOSIS

Definition

An acquired stricture or narrowing of the external auditory canal (Fig. 7.31), most commonly occurring in the region of the isthmus.

Aetiology

Canal stenosis may develop as the result of trauma to the skin of the external auditory canal. The trauma may be the result of an accidental laceration, chronic self-manipulation, chronic otitis externa and, on rare occasions, following the use of instruments in the external canal in cases of keratosis obturans. Once the skin lining the external canal has been lacerated, exuberant granulations within the external canal may epithelialize, producing a resultant skin-covered fibrous tissue stenosis.

Symptoms

There are usually no symptoms unless there is an accumulation of wax and debris medial to the stenosis, causing a conductive hearing loss.

Otoscopic appearances

The stricture occurs most commonly in the narrowest portion of the external canal (the isthmus). The stricture may be wide enough to allow migration of the epithelium from the deep canal to the outside to occur normally (Fig. 7.31). In some cases, the lumen may be reduced to a tiny pinhole (Fig. 7.32) behind which desquamated keratin may be trapped.

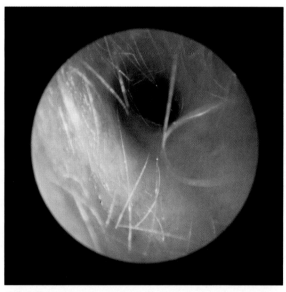

Fig. 7.31   External canal stenosis. This patient developed a canal stenosis at the isthmus following removal of keratosis obturans and debridement of granulation tissue. The membranous stenosis is seen at the isthmus and the actual lumen of the canal has been narrowed to approximately 4 mm in diameter.

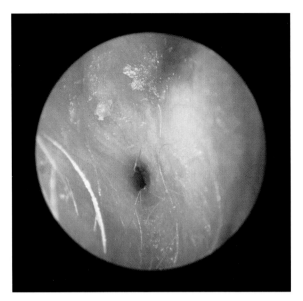

Fig. 7.32 External canal stenosis. The lumen of the deep canal in this patient has been narrowed to a pinpoint as the result of recurring episodes of otitis externa.

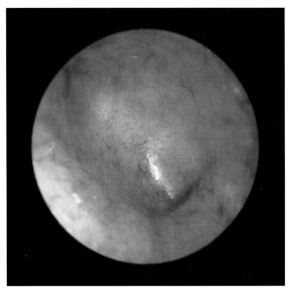

Fig. 7.33 False fundus. The false fundus is seen as an abnormally thick membrane resembling skin located at the isthmus of the external auditory canal.

Treatment guidelines

When the stenosis is responsible for the accumulation of wax or keratin debris in the medial portion of the canal, surgical excision may be indicated (Fig. 7.32). This condition, at its most extreme, may cause a total occlusion of the external canal (a false fundus).

FALSE FUNDUS

Definition

In this acquired condition, the external auditory canal ends blindly at the bony cartilaginous junction (Fig. 7.33).

Aetiology

A false fundus may develop following a severe injury to the epithelium lining the external ear canal: it occurs if granulation tissue is produced at the isthmus in such quantity that it totally occludes the ear canal and then becomes epithelialized.

Symptoms

The patient usually has a severe conductive hearing loss.

Otoscopic appearances

A false fundus is usually recognized when the end of the external canal is closer to the speculum during otoscopic examination than the examiner would normally anticipate. The false fundus also lacks the normal anatomical landmarks of the tympanic membrane, in particular the handle of the malleus (Fig. 7.33). Frequently, the fundus shows an abnormal thickness resembling skin, as compared to the normal translucency of a tympanic membrane, or it takes on a characteristic magenta hue.

Further investigations

A computerized tomography scan of the external canal and middle ear is required to determine exactly the location of the false fundus and to assess whether or not there is an underlying cholesteatoma.

Treatment guidelines

These patients should be referred for a specialist assessment, since there is the possibility of entrapped epithelium behind the false fundus, resulting in the development of a cholesteatoma.

MALIGNANT OTITIS EXTERNA

Definition

A severe and aggressive erosive form of otitis externa which occurs in elderly diabetics and otherwise immunocompromised patients. This condition is frequently fatal unless recognized and energetically treated at an early stage. Malignant otitis externa is not malignant in the sense of neoplasia, but is potentially lethal due to the fulminating spread of infection which may involve bone, cranial nerves and the cranial contents. A better descriptive title for this condition would be 'potentially fatal otitis externa'!

Aetiology

The causative organism is *Pseudomonas aeruginosa*, which is invariably found; the patient is almost always either diabetic or a severely immunocompromised individual. In these patients there appears to be a defect in the immune defence system which would normally limit the invasive capability of this bacterium.

Symptoms

The initial symptoms are those of an acute otitis externa, with local pain and discharge from the ear canal. As the infection progresses, the pain becomes quite severe and unremitting, and cranial nerve palsy may appear.

Malignant otitis externa is characterized by the progressive spread of infection from the ear canal into the adjacent structures. Frequently, the infection will spread into the temporal bone, causing osteomyelitis which may extend to the base of the skull, resulting in multiple cranial nerve palsies, meningitis, brain abscess or death.

Otoscopic appearances

The meatus is filled with a purulent discharge. The hallmark of malignant otitis externa is an area of infected granulation tissue on the floor of the cartilaginous ear canal near the junction between the cartilaginous and bony portions of the canal (Fig. 7.34). If the granulation tissue is removed, a defect may be found tracking under the bony external canal. The underlying skin is swollen and granulation tissue is often present within the external canal, arising from the junction of the bony and cartilaginous portions.

Further investigations

It is critical that this malignant otitis externa is diagnosed at an early stage so that appropriate treatment can be initiated before the osteomyelitis has spread beyond the possibility of treatment. The first step towards the correct diagnosis is *clinical suspicion* (i.e. severe otitis externa in a diabetic or immunocompromised individual). A gallium scan should then be done. Gallium 67 citrate will show the infected focus in the involved temporal bone by binding to the granulocytes (Fig. 7.35). Urinalysis and a blood sugar level should be carried out in any elderly patient with refractory otitis externa, especially if *Pseudomonas* has been cultured.

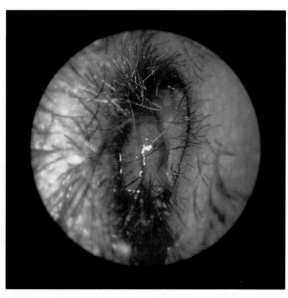

Fig. 7.34   Malignant otitis externa. Granulation tissue with a mucoid exudate is seen arising from the junction between the bony and cartilaginous portions of the canal.

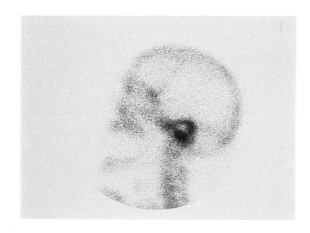

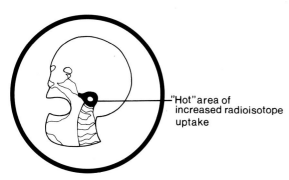

—"Hot" area of increased radioisotope uptake

Fig. 7.35 Malignant otitis externa. Note the 'hot' area of isotope uptake around the external auditory canal in this gallium scan of a patient with malignant otitis externa.

Treatment guidelines

In malignant otitis externa, simple aural toilet followed by the application of topical antibiotic drops are *ineffective measures*. These patients require urgent referral for a specialist opinion and admission to hospital. The initial treatment includes scrupulous debridement of the ear, using the operating microscope, and an adequate course of both systemic and topical antibiotics which are effective against *Pseudomonas*. The oral administration of a non-steroidal anti-inflammatory preparation such as indomethacin may also be of substantial value. If an aminoglycoside antibiotic is used, serum levels and renal function should be carefully monitored

to avoid possible ototoxicity and nephrotoxicity. Hyperbaric oxygen therapy may be of benefit as an adjunct to antibiotic treatment.

When medical treatment is unsuccessful, a wide surgical excision of the involved necrotic tissue is indicated. This may include removal of the pinna or even extirpation of a large part of the temporal bone.

HERPES ZOSTER OTICUS (SYNONYMS: RAMSAY HUNT SYNDROME, GENICULATE HERPES)

Herpes zoster oticus is an infection of the geniculate ganglion (seventh cranial nerve), characterized by a vesicular eruption of the skin of the external ear. It may occur in varying degrees of severity: herpes auricularis, an isolated herpes infection of the skin of the external ear canal and pinna; herpes auricularis with facial palsy and herpes auricularis with facial palsy and involvement of the eighth cranial nerve causing hearing loss and/or loss of balance. This condition may also be associated with a herpes infection of the upper cervical roots or the glossopharyngeal nerve, the latter producing vesicles on the soft palate.

Aetiology

The causative organism is the herpes zoster virus, which is also responsible for chickenpox.

Symptoms

Initially the patient experiences a hot feeling within the ear, which develops into pain of increasing severity. Malaise may be present in the early stages. Hearing loss, tinnitus or giddiness may be present when the inner ear is involved. Long after the infection has resolved, many patients continue to suffer severe pain in the previously involved area (post-herpetic pain).

Otoscopic appearances

The vesicles may appear on the superficial pinna within the conchal bowl (Fig. 7.36), along the skin of the external canal and sometimes even on the tympanic membrane (Fig. 7.37).

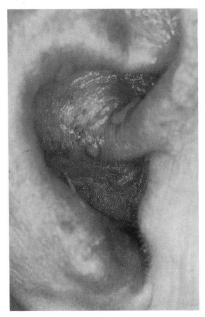

Fig. 7.36 Herpes zoster oticus. Numerous crusted vesicles are seen scattered throughout the conchal bowl.

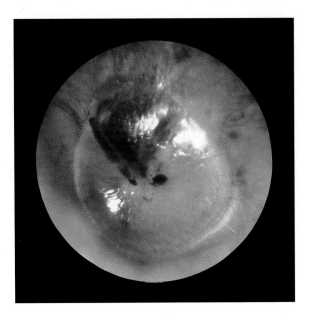

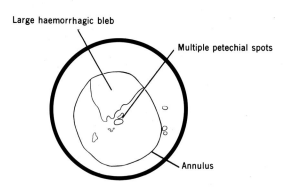

Fig. 7.37 Tympanic herpes zoster. This is the same patient as shown in Figure 7.36. A haemorrhagic bleb is present on the tympanic membrane overlying the short process of the malleus.

Further investigations

A pure tone audiogram should be done to determine whether there has been involvement of the cochlear portion of the inner ear. Tests of vestibular function may be required if there are signs or symptoms, such as nystagmus or vertigo, suggesting vestibular involvement. The eye should be carefully examined to ensure that the patient is not developing a herpes infection of the eye.

Tympanometry with measurement of the stapedial reflexes is useful in localizing the lesion in those cases where the facial nerve is involved (after the canal has healed).

Treatment guidelines

The patient should be started immediately on a course of oral acyclovir. Topical acyclovir ointment should also be applied to the cutaneous lesions. The vesicles should be kept dry and an oral antipruritic such as an antihistamine administered to prevent scratching and subsequent secondary infection.

In those cases in which a total facial nerve paralysis has occurred, the use of oral prednisone in high doses is sometimes beneficial. Steroids may also be used to prevent subsequent post-herpetic neuralgia. Complete recovery of facial nerve function is less common than with Bell's palsy. Some surgeons advocate surgical decompression of the facial nerve up to and including the internal auditory canal.

SQUAMOUS CELL CARCINOMA OF THE EXTERNAL AUDITORY CANAL (SYNONYMS: SQUAMOUS EPITHELIOMA, EPIDERMOID CARCINOMA)

Definition

A malignant neoplasm arising from the stratified squamous epithelial layer of the external auditory canal.

Aetiology

Squamous cell carcinoma of the external ear canal is associated with chronic otorrhoea in 75% of cases, suggesting that chronic infection or irritation may be a significant aetiological factor. It should be noted, however, that this is an extremely rare complication of chronic ear disease.

Symptoms

The most suspicious symptoms are *bleeding* from the external canal and chronic otorrhoea which has recently become associated with *pain*.

Otoscopic appearances

An early carcinoma may form an ulcer in the skin of the external canal or may appear as a small area of granulation tissue. A large polypoid tumour can totally occlude the external canal (Fig. 7.38). It should, however, be emphasized that there are no absolute otoscopic signs which are truly diagnostic of malignant tumours of the external auditory canal (Fig. 7.39). Any unusual or uncharacteristic growths arising in the external canal should be biopsied.

Further investigations

All tissue removed from the external auditory canal should be submitted for histopathological sectioning, staining and microscopy. Occasionally, a squamous cell carcinoma is discovered unexpectedly after sending an apparently benign inflammatory polyp for routine histopathology.

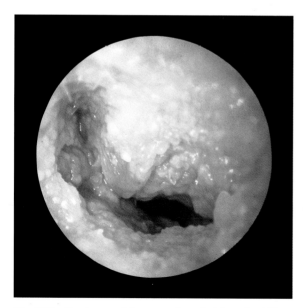

Fig. 7.38 Carcinoma of the external canal. A large knobbly growth is almost obliterating the external auditory canal. On biopsy this was shown to be a moderately well differentiated squamous cell carcinoma.

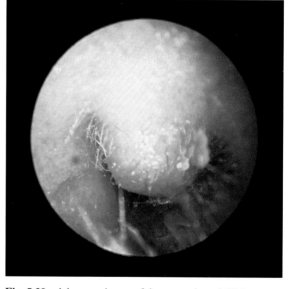

Fig. 7.39 Adenocarcinoma of the external canal. This apparently innocent soft tissue lesion arising from the posterosuperior wall of the cartilaginous external canal was excised solely on the basis of the clinician's inability to diagnose the lesion otoscopically. Pathological examination revealed the lesion to be a primary adenocarcinoma of the external canal.

If *pain or bleeding* develops in cases of chronic otitis externa or chronic suppurative otitis media, a careful inspection of the ear must be carried out to exclude the possibility of an underlying neoplasm. A computerized tomography scan is useful in determining the extent and spread of malignant lesions in this area.

Treatment guidelines

These cases should be referred promptly to a specialist for management.

OTHER MALIGNANT DISORDERS

Melanomata and malignant growths arising from the glands of the external ear canal (ceruminoma, adenocarcinoma) may also occur. It is important to differentiate malignant canal disease primarily involving the external auditory canal from that which encroaches upon it, as for example carcinoma of the middle ear, parotid tumours, or rodent ulcer of the pinna.

8. Diseases of the tympanic membrane and middle ear

THE NORMAL TYMPANIC MEMBRANE

The normal tympanic membrane (Figs 8.1 and 8.2) is a pale, grey, ovoid, semi-transparent membrane which is set obliquely at the medial end of the bony external auditory canal. The anterior margin (*anterior recess*) of the tympanic membrane may be difficult to see otoscopically if the normal convex curvature of the anterior bony canal is especially marked (Fig. 8.3).

Part of the most lateral of the three ossicles, the handle of the malleus, is visible extending downwards and backwards, with a spatulated end (the *umbo*), which sits at the apex of the triangular *cone of light*. The lateral process of the malleus is seen as a small prominent white protuberance arising from the upper end of the malleus handle.

The cone of light is a band of light which is reflected back down the canal by the only portion of the tympanic membrane which is truly at right-angles to the central axis of the external auditory canal. Clinically, the cone of light is seen as a triangular brightly illuminated area on the tympanic membrane which extends anteroinferiorly from the umbo of a normal tympanic membrane.

The *pars flaccida* (Shrapnell's membrane; Fig. 8.1) is divided from the *pars tensa* by the anterior and posterior malleolar folds, which curve like a pair of wings from the region of the lateral process of the malleus. The long process of the incus and its articulation with the head of the stapes and the chorda tympani nerve passing between the handle of the malleus and the long process of the incus may frequently be seen

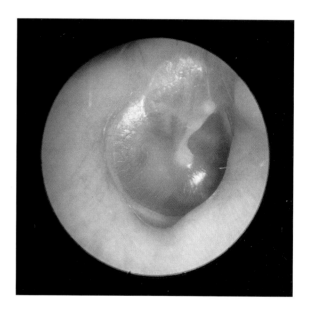

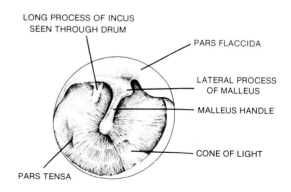

LONG PROCESS OF INCUS SEEN THROUGH DRUM

PARS FLACCIDA

LATERAL PROCESS OF MALLEUS

MALLEUS HANDLE

CONE OF LIGHT

PARS TENSA

Fig. 8.1 A thin normal right tympanic membrane. Note the malleus, the chorda tympani nerve and the long process of the incus. The latter two can be seen through the posterosuperior quadrant of this very thin and transparent tympanic membrane. This tympanic membrane has an unusually prominent pars flaccida.

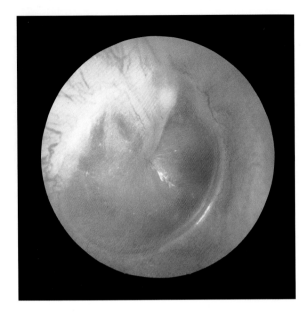

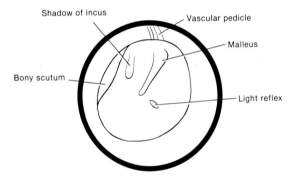

Fig. 8.2 Normal tympanic membrane. This picture shows the more usual appearance of a normal (right) tympanic membrane. Note the thin plate of bone (the scutum) covering the chorda tympani nerve and the vascular leash posterior to the malleus.

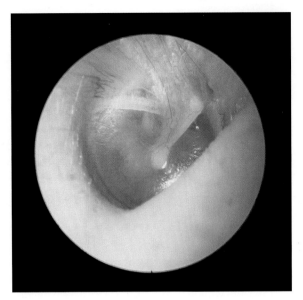

Fig. 8.3 A thin normal right tympanic membrane. The chorda tympani nerve and the long process of the incus are clearly visible. Note how the anteroinferior aspect of the tympanic membrane (the anterior sulcus) is hidden behind the posterior curvature of the anteroinferior bony canal.

through the posterosuperior quadrant of the pars tensa of a thin tympanic membrane.

THE RED REFLEX

Mechanical stimulation of the skin of the external canal by the insertion of a speculum may cause a reflex dilatation of the circumferential and manubrial blood vessels supplying the tympanic membrane (Figs 8.4 and 8.5). Following a prolonged examination of the ear, this vasodilatation may produce an appearance mimicking that of an early acute otitis media. It

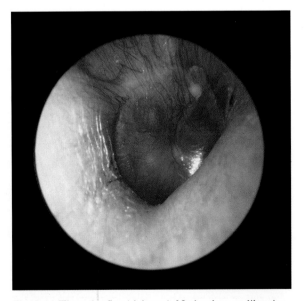

Fig. 8.4 The red reflex (right ear). Notice the vasodilatation of the vessels running along the handle of the malleus and over the roof of the canal. The tympanic membrane is normal and does not show any swelling or abnormal vascularity. This vascular reflex is a normal response to instrumentation in the canal.

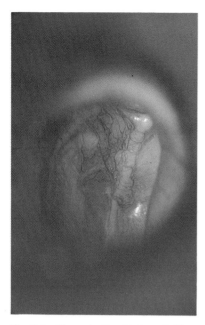

Fig. 8.5 The red reflex (right ear). The tiny dilated blood vessels along the handle of the malleus can be seen more clearly under higher magnification.

is important to note that the radial vessels do not become dilated in this type of reflex vasodilatation; this differentiates the red reflex from acute otitis media. A similar appearance is produced by any form of physical stimulation of the skin lining the external auditory canal, e.g. after the removal of wax by curetting, suction, syringing, or after caloric testing. This reflex vasodilatation appears to result from mechanical stimulation of the cutaneous nerves supplying the skin of the external auditory canal.

TRAUMATIC PERFORATIONS OF THE TYMPANIC MEMBRANE

Traumatic perforations of the tympanic membrane may result either from violent changes in the air pressure within the external auditory canal and middle ear (e.g. from a slap on the ear or as the result of an explosion) or from direct solid body trauma to the tympanic membrane (e.g. the insertion of cotton-tipped applicators, bobby pins, matchsticks, etc.). Traumatic perforations rarely follow forceful

syringing, unless the tympanic membrane has already been weakened by previous disease.

Symptoms
Pain, bleeding, hearing loss, tinnitus and occasionally severe vertigo of sudden onset may be present.

Otoscopic appearances
Those injuries which result from sudden pressure changes within the external canal usually produce perforations of the anteroinferior quadrant (Figs 8.6–8.8). This type of perforation characteristically has everted ragged edges, since the initial positive pressure wave is followed by a high negative wave which flips the margins of the perforation laterally. Ossicular damage is rare in this type of perforation; however, there is sometimes a severe temporary sensorineural hearing loss which results from the effects of the violent pressure change upon the cochlea.

By contrast, those perforations which result from the insertion of foreign materials into the ear canal (direct trauma) tend to occur posteriorly (Fig. 8.9), since this is the most directly accessible aspect of the tympanic membrane. These perforations are often associated with ossicular damage, since both the incus and its articulation with the stapes are at risk behind the posterosuperior quadrant of the tympanic membrane. The edges of the perforation may be haemorrhagic and fresh blood may be seen in the deep meatus. The subsequent appearance of a purulent discharge indicates that a secondary infection has developed.

Further investigations
Because of the possibility of damage to the ossicular chain or cochlea, an assessment of hearing using both tuning forks and pure tone audiometry is necessary. This is especially important in those cases which may have medicolegal implications.

In those cases caused by the detonation of an explosive device, the implosive force, in addition to causing a perforation of the tympanic membrane, may also in rare cases be conducted through the perilymph producing a rupture of the round window membrane. In this event, a

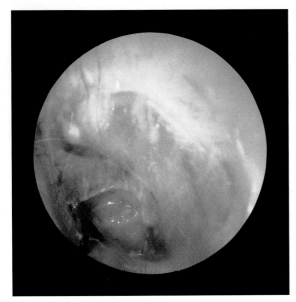

Fig. 8.6 Traumatic anterior perforation (left ear). Notice in the 6 o'clock position the moderately large anteroinferior perforation which has resulted from a slap on the patient's left ear. A small haematoma is seen underneath the handle of the malleus. The everted edge of the flap (seen anteriorly) is characteristic of a traumatic perforation.

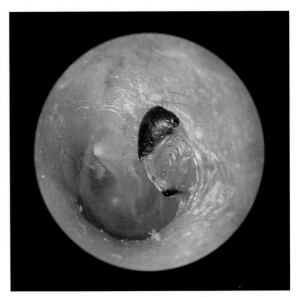

Fig. 8.8 Healed traumatic central perforation. This is the ear of the patient shown in Figure 8.6, 1 month after the injury. The perforation has healed and the scab under which the healing occurred has been carried off the tympanic membrane on to the skin of the bony canal (at 2 o'clock position) by the normal migratory process of the epithelium lining the external canal.

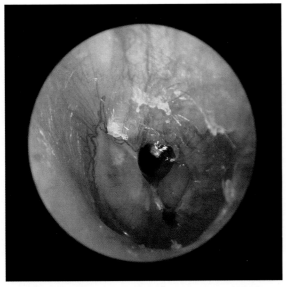

Fig. 8.7 Traumatic central perforation (left ear). Notice the central traumatic perforation which was the result of a violent slap on the ear 3 days previously.

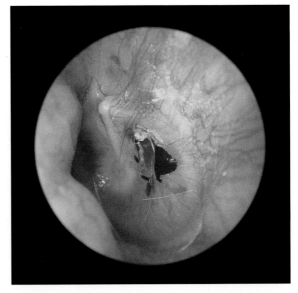

Fig. 8.9 Traumatic posterosuperior perforation (left ear). This patient accidently stuck a twig into her left ear. Injuries of the posterosuperior quadrant are potentially serious because of the risk of damage to the long process of the incus and the stapes which underly this area.

profound sensorineural hearing loss occurs, usually accompanied by vertigo and nystagmus. This may also occur after direct trauma to the oval window.

Therapeutic guidelines

The ear canal should be kept clean and dry to prevent secondary infection. Topical and systemic antibiotics are best withheld unless there is a strong possibility of secondary infection occurring, e.g. after the entry of water into the middle ear.

Most (85–95%) small and medium size perforations will heal spontaneously within 3 months. Large perforations and those which involve the annulus may require surgical closure; however, this is usually not carried out for some months and then only if spontaneous healing does not occur.

OTITIC BAROTRAUMA (AEROTITIS MEDIA)

Definition

Damage to the middle ear cleft caused by a failure of the eustachian tube to equalize the difference between intratympanic and atmospheric pressure.

Aetiology

Otitic barotrauma usually occurs when the atmospheric pressure is significantly higher than the pressure within the middle ear cleft and when eustachian tube function is inadequate, e.g. during descent in an aircraft, or during diving either in water or in a compression chamber.

Symptoms

The symptoms are variable but commonly ear pain, hearing loss, tinnitus and woolliness are experienced. The presence of fluid within the middle ear may present as a 'swishing' sensation, brought about by head movement.

Otoscopic appearances

The otoscopic appearances of otitic barotrauma are variable and include erythema of the tympanic membrane, solitary or multiple

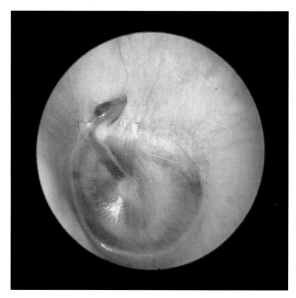

Fig. 8.10 Otitic barotrauma (left ear). This patient went flying while suffering from an acute viral upper respiratory infection. During descent he was unable to equalize the pressure changes in his middle ear and consequently suffered an earache. Three days later, the linear interstitial haemorrhages along the handle of the malleus provide visible evidence of previous barotrauma.

interstitial haemorrhage of the tympanic membrane (Fig. 8.10), often with streaking in patches in the pars flaccida and along the sides of the handle of the malleus (Fig. 8.11), a golden-yellow serous exudate (Fig. 8.12) or even a frank haemotympanum. Although rarely associated with flying and diving, a rupture of the tympanic membrane can occur following violent pressure changes.

Further investigations

The hearing should be tested, to ensure that the cochlea has not been damaged.

Round window membrane rupture and fistula

As a result of sudden onset of negative middle ear pressure, a rupture of the round window membrane can occur, resulting in a leakage of perilymph into the middle ear. This produces a sudden and often severe sensorineural hearing loss, with or without associated vertigo and nystagmus. In some cases, the sensorineural hearing loss may fluctuate.

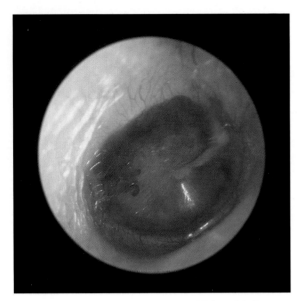

Fig. 8.11   Otitic barotrauma (right ear). This patient has developed a larger interstitial haemorrhage under the posterosuperior quadrant of the tympanic membrane.

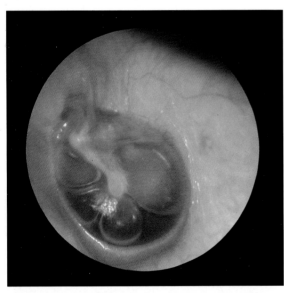

Fig. 8.12   Otitic barotrauma (left ear). This patient was unable to clear her ears during descent in an aircraft. She has developed a serous effusion which is visible within the middle ear. There is an air–fluid level extending on either side of the malleus, as well as a small central bubble of air within the golden-yellow effusion inferiorly: the upper part of the mesotympanum is aerated.

The possibility of a round window membrane rupture should be considered if during the Weber test the tuning fork is heard in the unaffected ear, indicating the presence of a sensorineural hearing loss in the affected ear. In this case, the patient should be immediately referred to an otologist for management. If strict bedrest with the affected ear uppermost fails to restore hearing within a few days, an exploratory tympanotomy to identify and seal the round window (perilymph) fistula is then indicated.

Therapeutic guidelines

Otitic barotrauma can usually be prevented by avoiding air travel during upper respiratory tract infections. If this is impossible, the use of a topical nasal decongestant drop (e.g. xylometazoline hydrochloride 0.1%) and oral systemic decongestants combined with regular autoinflation by Valsalva manoeuvre during descent are helpful measures.

The effects of established barotrauma will usually resolve spontaneously within 6 weeks. Treatment with topical and systemic nasal decongestants is useful to restore eustachian tube function and normal middle ear pressure. If necessary, the middle ear can be aspirated and ventilated through a myringotomy.

If travelling is essential during an acute respiratory infection in a patient with a history of barotrauma, then it may be prudent to insert ventilation tubes prophylactically prior to the flight. Similar needs may arise with train or car trips through mountainous areas.

HAEMOTYMPANUM

Definition

The presence of extravasated blood or blood-stained fluid behind the tympanic membrane in the middle ear space.

Aetiology

A heamotympanum may develop following barotrauma, head injury, temporal bone fracture, or in association with secretory otitis media.

Symptoms

The symptoms are those of the causative disease

and may include hearing loss, a feeling of pressure, fullness or pain.

Otoscopic appearances

When bleeding is confined to the tympanic membrane, as after barotrauma induced by flying or diving, bright red streaks appear in the tympanic membrane.

In the classical haemotympanum, the middle ear fills with blood and the tympanic membrane assumes a uniform bright red, dark red, brown, or gun-metal blue coloration depending upon the colour of the bloody fluid within the middle ear (Fig. 8.13). In long-standing cases of haemotympanum, degradation of the haemoglobin occurs and a dark-brown coloration results (*chocolate ear drum*; Fig. 8.14). Frequently, when aspirated the fluid is found to consist of reddish, brownish or bluish thick mucus (Fig. 8.15).

Further investigations

Follow-up audiometry should be carried out after resolution of the haemotympanum.

Therapeutic guidelines

The treatment of haemotympanum is essentially that of the underlying cause. The haemotympanum will usually resolve spontaneously. If resolution does not occur, the fluid may be drained through a myringotomy.

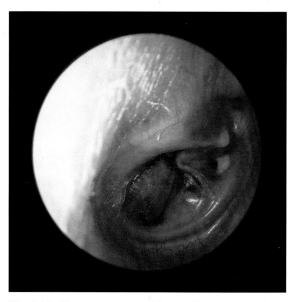

Fig. 8.14 Haemotympanum (right ear). The dark purple colour of this patient's tympanic membrane is caused by a very dark brown mucoid fluid which resulted from a severe viral otitis media.

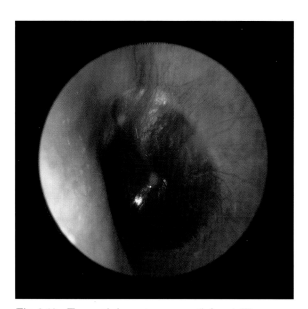

Fig. 8.13 Traumatic haemotympanum (left ear). The middle ear of this patient has filled with blood from a recent skull fracture. Notice how the fresh blood within the middle ear gives the tympanic membrane a dark red colour.

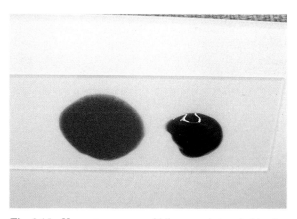

Fig. 8.15 Haemotympanum middle ear aspirates. As blood within the middle ear undergoes degeneration it changes from a bright red colour (**left**) to a dark brown (**right**).

TEMPORAL BONE FRACTURES

Definition
A fracture within the temporal bone.

Aetiology
A head injury may result in a fracture of the temporal bone. Longitudinal fractures of the temporal bone—the most common—often run through the roof of the middle ear (the tegmen tympani), causing a haemotympanum. Less commonly, disruption of the tympanic membrane may occur, with resultant bleeding into the external canal. The bony annulus may occasionally be fractured. Backward displacement of the condyle of the mandible from a blow to the chin may also cause a fracture of the anterior wall of the bony external canal.

Otoscopic appearances
The tell-tale sign of a temporal bone fracture is a deformity of the annulus or bony canal wall resulting from the displaced fragments of bone (Fig. 8.16).

Temporal bone fractures heal by fibrous union, and long after the original injury, the tell-tale sign of a fracture line may still be visible otoscopically, usually on the posterosuperior canal wall near the annulus.

Further investigations
If a watery discharge persists, with or without blood tinging, the possibility of a cerebrospinal fluid leak (CSF otorrhoea) should be considered. Appropriate radiological studies, including a high-resolution computerized tomography scan and emission studies with radiopharmaceuticals, will be required and follow-up audiometry should be carried out.

Therapeutic guidelines
The management of any temporal bone fracture is always secondary to the treatment of the underlying head injury and is essentially expectant with frequent re-examinations and pure tone audiometric follow-up.

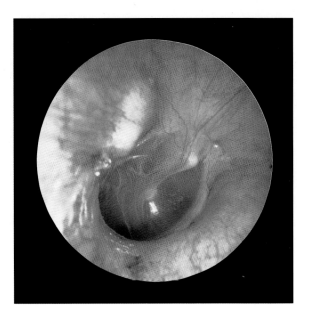

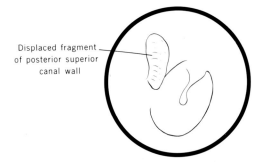

Displaced fragment of posterior superior canal wall

Fig. 8.16   Temporal bone fracture (right ear). In this patient a portion of the posterosuperior canal wall has been displaced and remains as a tell-tale clue to the previous temporal bone fracture.

BULLOUS MYRINGITIS (OTITIS EXTERNA HAEMORRHAGICA, MYRINGITIS BULLOSA)

Definition
A distinctive form of otitis externa, characterized by the appearance of fluid-filled haemorrhagic blebs on the tympanic membrane and skin of the deep external meatus.

Aetiology
While the exact causative agent responsible for bullous myringitis has yet to be conclusively

identified, both the influenzal viruses and *Mycoplasma pneumonia* are suspect.

Symptoms

Severe local pain within the ear is usually the first symptom and may be followed by the spontaneous appearance of a blood-tinged serous or serosanguineous discharge. A conductive deafness may occur from swelling of the skin of the external canal or from the development of a secondary serous otitis media. In a small number of cases, inner ear involvement with sensorineural hearing loss and vertigo may occur. Occasionally, viral encephalitis is associated with this condition.

Otoscopic appearances

The tympanic membrane is covered by multiple blebs (blisters) filled either with a serous (Fig. 8.17) or a serosanguineous fluid (Fig. 8.18). Petechial haemorrhages are commonly seen in the skin around the base of the blebs (Fig. 8.19). If the blebs become confluent, it may be difficult to distinguish this condition from an acute otitis media.

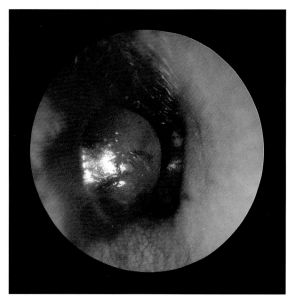

Fig. 8.18 Bullous myringitis (right ear). Notice the large bleb overlying the posterior canal wall. It contains a serous effusion with a small collection of blood in the inferior portion.

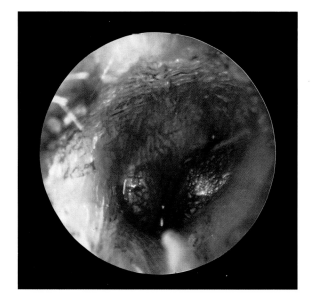

Fig. 8.17 Bullous myringitis (right ear). Note the two large haemorrhagic bullae present over the inferior two-thirds of the tympanic membrane. The bulla on the right extends on to the skin of the bony canal.

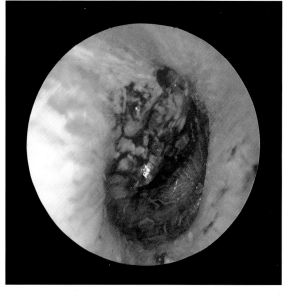

Fig. 8.19 Bullous myringitis after puncture. This is the same patient as shown in Figure 8.18. The bleb has been punctured and the tympanic membrane is now visible. The middle ear contained a small quantity of serous fluid.

Therapeutic guidelines

Since there is no specific treatment for the causative organism, therapy is directed towards adequate analgesia and the prevention of secondary infection by keeping the ear clean and dry.

GRANULAR MYRINGITIS

Definition

Chronic inflammation of the external surface of the tympanic membrane associated with an ulceration of the outer epithelial layer of the tympanic membrane and the production of granulation tissue.

Aetiology

An ulceration in the outer epithelial surface of the tympanic membrane may occasionally develop as a complication of otitis externa. When the outer epithelial layer of the tympanic membrane has been destroyed by the inflammatory process, the fibrous layer is exposed and may become covered with granulation tissue.

Symptoms

Painless mucopurulent otorrhoea is the most common symptom; however, all the other symptoms of chronic otitis externa may also be present.

Otoscopic appearances

Granular myringitis may present as one of two different forms: localized or diffuse granular myringitis. In localized granular myringitis, localized areas of bright red granulation tissue will be seen arising from the lateral surface of the tympanic membrane (Fig. 8.20). In more diffuse granular myringitis, the entire surface of the tympanic membrane has an erythematous granular appearance (Fig. 8.21).

Further investigations

A swab of any discharge within the canal should be sent for bacterial and fungal culture in order to identify any pathogens present within the canal.

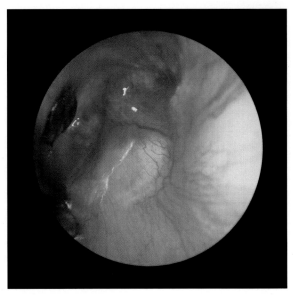

Fig. 8.20 Localized granular myringitis (right ear). There is a localized mass of exuberant granulation tissue arising from the tympanic membrane over its inferior half. Notice also the diffuse exostoses of the canal.

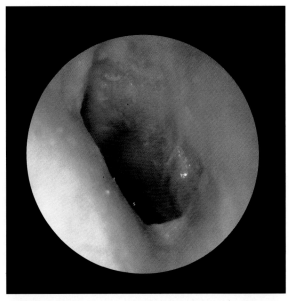

Fig. 8.21 Diffuse granular myringitis (left ear). In this patient the entire tympanic membrane is covered with granulation tissue.

Treatment guidelines

Granular myringitis is an extremely difficult condition to treat and, if the appropriate topical steroid-containing antibacterial or antifungal preparations do not produce resolution, then surgical removal of the granulations may be necessary.

ACUTE OTITIS MEDIA

Definition

An acute suppurative infection of the mucosal lining of the middle ear cleft. The middle ear cleft includes the eustachian tube, tympanic cavity, mastoid antrum and mastoid air cells.

Aetiology

The causative organisms most commonly encountered include *Staphylococcus aureus*, haemolytic *Streptococcus*, *Pneumococcus* and *Haemophilus influenzae*, which is the most common pathogen in children. These micro-organisms usually reach the middle ear by ascending the eustachian tube from the nasopharynx, frequently following a viral upper respiratory tract infection, which damages the local defence mechanisms.

While the progression of acute otitis media has classically been divided into a series of stages, each with different symptoms and otoscopic appearances, in practice this disease usually progresses rapidly, with no clearly separated staging.

The stage of eustachian tube obstruction

Symptoms
Initially a mild hearing loss with a stuffy feeling in the ear or slight pain may be the only complaint. In children this stage is often silent.

Otoscopic appearances
The earliest clinical sign seen in acute otitis media consists of redness and swelling in the pars flaccida (Fig. 8.22). The tympanic membrane is retracted and the malleus handle assumes a more horizontal position, with the lateral process appearing more prominent. The normal lustre of the tympanic membrane is lost.

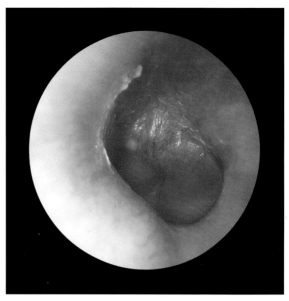

Fig. 8.22 Acute otitis media—the stage of redness (right ear). Note the erythema, oedema and slight outward bulging of the pars flaccida. This is the earliest clinical sign of acute otitis media.

The stage of redness

Symptoms
At this stage there is increasing earache and hearing loss. Systemic symptoms are now usually present, including fever, nausea, vomiting and abdominal pain or diarrhoea in children.

Otoscopic appearances
The manubrial and circumferential vessels supplying the tympanic membrane dilate and the entire tympanic membrane eventually becomes uniformly fiery red in colour.

The stage of suppuration (Fig. 8.23)

Symptoms
The pain is often excruciating at this stage and the systemic symptoms increase in severity.

Otoscopic appearances
In severe or untreated cases, creamy-white pus forms under pressure within the middle ear and

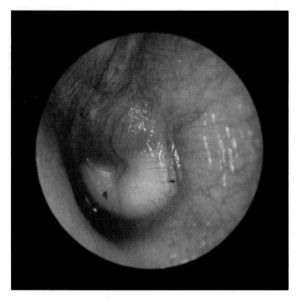

Fig. 8.23   Acute otitis media—the stage of suppuration (left ear). The tympanic membrane is bulging outwards as a creamy-white mucopurulent exudate fills the lower two-thirds of the middle ear.

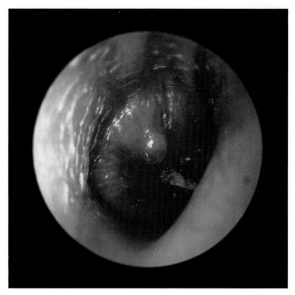

Fig. 8.24   Acute otitis media—later in the stage of suppuration (right ear). In severe cases of acute otitis media, the bacterial infection within the middle ear may spread directly into the tympanic membrane, causing necrosis of the radial vessels and bleeding from these vessels into the fibrous middle layer of the drum. Note the linear streaks of interstitial haemorrhage present around the umbo. Note also the central 'herniated' area where the strength-providing fibrous middle layer has become necrotic, allowing the outer epithelial layer to herniate outwards.

the tympanic membrane bulges outwards. The posterosuperior portion of the tympanic membrane becomes especially prominent.

This increasing intratympanic pressure causes the tympanic membrane to become oedematous and much of the pain seems to be due to local infection and ischaemia within the drum.

The bacterial infection within the middle ear may spread directly into the tympanic membrane, causing initially necrosis and rupture of the radial blood vessels. Rupture of the radial vessels appears as haemorrhagic patches in the tympanic membrane (Fig. 8.24).

Prior to bursting, the drum is greyish at the point of rupture, indicating ischaemic necrosis of the fibrous middle layer (Fig. 8.25). The tympanic membrane, at this stage, can be considered as the outer wall of an abscess cavity. It ulcerates on the inner surface, perforating to allow drainage of the abscess with relief of pain.

Healing of the perforation usually occurs after the infection has resolved.

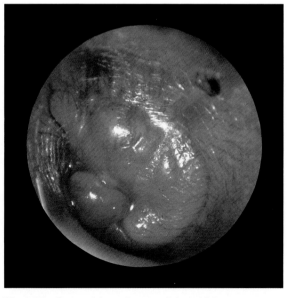

Fig. 8.25   Acute otitis media—much later in the stage of suppuration (left ear). The tympanic membrane is now bulging severely and about to perforate.

The stage of resolution

Symptoms

After the tympanic membrane has ruptured, the ear becomes less painful and otorrhoea is the principal complaint.

Otoscopic appearances

A small perforation in an inflamed tympanic membrane is seen, often with a bead of pus coming from it (Fig. 8.26), together with pus in the external canal. Resolution slowly occurs and the tympanic membrane will normally heal spontaneously in a few days. The tympanic membrane does not assume a fully normal appearance for approximately 6 weeks after the onset of an attack of acute otitis media.

Further investigations

In cases of acute otitis media, a swab from the nasopharynx or a sample of any discharge present in the external canal should be sent for

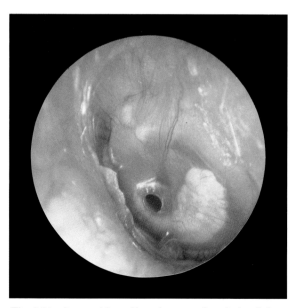

Fig. 8.26 Acute otitis media—the stage of resolution (left ear). The bacterial infection within the middle ear has drained from a small anteroinferior perforation and the tympanic membrane has now returned to a non-inflamed state. Notice the large patch of tympanosclerosis present in the posteroinferior quadrant.

bacterial culture, to identify the causative organism and establish its antibiotic sensitivity.

Therapeutic guidelines

The primary aim of treatment is to alter the natural history of this disease, thereby preventing the production of pus under pressure and avoiding subsequent complications such as acute mastoiditis, meningitis or brain abscess.

The approach to treatment will depend upon the stage at which the disease is seen. In the early case, the use of topical and systemic nasal decongestants to assist in re-opening the eustachian tube is of some value. An adequate dose of an appropriate antibiotic should be administered promptly. While penicillin V is usually adequate for adults, amoxycillin is indicated in children in view of the likelihood of *Haemophilus influenzae* being the causative organism.

With the increasing frequency of beta-lactamase (penicillinase)-producing strains of *H. influenzae* and *Branhamella catarrhalis*, the possibility that these antibiotics may be inactivated by beta-lactamase should be considered. The recent development of a combination of amoxycillin and potassium clavulanate allows the successful use of amoxycillin in the presence of beta-lactamase-producing organisms. Potassium clavulanate is a chemical compound which is metabolized to produce clavulanic acid, which binds irreversibly to a wide range of beta-lactamase enzymes, rendering them inactive.

Systemic analgesics should be administered according to the requirements of the patient.

If the tympanic membrane is fiery red and obviously bulging due to the presence of pus under pressure, a carefully performed myringotomy will relieve pain by reducing oedema and draining the purulent contents of the middle ear into the external canal. In a co-operative patient, anaesthesia is not required if a sharp myringotome is used. A sample of the discharge should be cultured.

If the tympanic membrane has already perforated spontaneously, the external canal should be cleaned by drymopping and a sample of the discharge cultured.

The key to the successful treatment of acute otitis media is to achieve adequate blood levels of an appropriate antibiotic at an early stage. The administration of a full course of an appropriate antibiotic for at least 5–7 days is necessary to prevent the development of mastoiditis.

ACUTE MASTOIDITIS

Acute mastoiditis is an acute infection of the bony walls and partition of the mastoid air cell system. The bony walls of the air cells eventually break down with the accumulation of pus within the temporal bone.

Aetiology

Acute mastoiditis is nowadays a relatively infrequent complication of acute suppurative otitis media and is a consequence of the extension of infection beyond the mucosal lining of the middle ear cleft. Inadequate, incomplete or inappropriate antibiotic therapy prescribed in the treatment of acute suppurative otitis media probably suppresses the infective process just enough to prevent spontaneous rupture of the tympanic membrane (nature's myringotomy). The infection then continues in a relatively asymptomatic manner and the presence of a developing coalescent mastoiditis is often hidden until it appears as a post-auricular, subperiosteal abscess or as a serious intracranial complication (brain abscess or purulent meningitis).

Symptoms

The symptoms may be minimal in masked or incompletely treated mastoiditis and consist only of lassitude and a low-grade fever associated with an elevated white blood cell count occurring 2–3 weeks after the onset of acute otitis media. When present, pain or tenderness is maximal over Macewen's triangle. This surface marking of the mastoid antrum can be palpated by placing a finger on to—not behind—the pinna, just posterior to the crus of the helix. Since firm pressure in this area tends to be uncomfortable in the normal state, it is wise to compare the ears. Pain may also radiate along the mastoid process and the mastoid tip is sometimes tender.

Otoscopic appearances

The tympanic membrane in mastoiditis is always abnormal in appearance (Fig. 8.27). In untreated cases it may be red and bulging and the posterosuperior external canal wall will be oedematous and displaced downwards by intratympanic pus. More commonly, however, the patient has been treated by antibiotics which alter the natural course of the disease, and the tympanic membrane may simply appear dull greyish, resembling a resolving otitis media.

Further investigations

The suspicion that mastoiditis has occurred is based on clinical findings of continuing low-grade fever, an abnormal tympanic membrane appearance, pain or swelling over the mastoid, and is confirmed radiographically. Mastoid X-rays will show cloudiness and destruction of the bony partitions between the individual mastoid air cells. A full series of mastoid X-rays is desirable; however, if only limited radiological facilities are available, a Towne's view (35° frontal–occipital) should be requested. This is the most useful view, since it allows a comparison

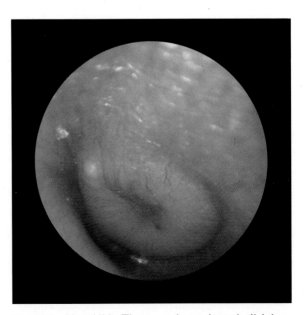

Fig. 8.27   Mastoiditis. The tympanic membrane is slightly bulging but not acutely inflamed (reddened). The diagnosis of mastoiditis cannot be made solely on the otoscopic appearance alone and X-rays are essential.

of both mastoid processes to be made. Today, the most accurate diagnostic test is a computerized tomography scan.

Therapeutic guidelines

In the absence of signs of pus under pressure, the initial treatment depends upon large doses of benzyl penicillin administered intramuscularly or intravenously.

If adequate antibiotic treatment does not lead to an improvement within 24 hours, a wide myringotomy should be made to establish drainage and to obtain a specimen for culture.

In those few cases in which the infection does not resolve, or in those presenting with a subperiosteal abscess or signs of intracranial infection, a cortical mastoidectomy is urgently required.

CASTS AND CRUSTS OF THE TYMPANIC MEMBRANE

Definition

A crust (Fig. 8.28) is a localized accumulation of corneocytes and dried inflammatory exudate located on the surface of the tympanic membrane. A cast (Fig. 8.29) is a crust which has become detached from the surface of the tympanic membrane.

Aetiology

Crust formation on the surface of the tympanic membrane is the result of a local infection of the tympanic membrane which occurs in some severe cases of acute otitis media when the infection within the middle ear spreads laterally into the tissues of the tympanic membrane. This localized infection produces a rapid accumulation of surface corneocytes into which a serous-like inflammatory exudate from the outer surface of the inflamed drum is absorbed.

Symptoms

Casts and crusts are generally asymptomatic. The observation of a crust on the surface of the tympanic membrane, or of a cast within the external canal, indicates that the patient has had a recent (within the past few weeks or months) episode of acute suppurative otitis media.

Otoscopic appearances

Clinically, tympanic membrane crusts are semi-translucent, golden-yellow in colour, and of a dry and brittle consistency (Fig. 8.28). Crusts

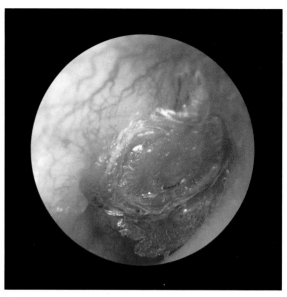

Fig. 8.28 Postacute otitis media—tympanic membrane crust (right ear). Note how the entire surface of the tympanic membrane is covered by a brittle golden-yellow crust.

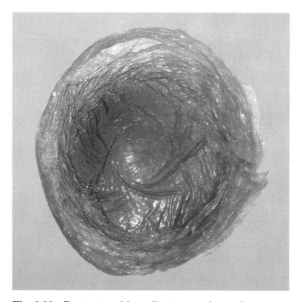

Fig. 8.29 Post acute otitis media—tympanic membrane cast. This round golden-yellow cast was removed from the external canal of an adult who had a severe episode of acute otitis media 2 months previously.

may vary in size from those covering only a small area of the tympanic membrane to those covering the entire membrane. The medial surface of a detached cast (Fig. 8.29) usually duplicates the surface contours of the underlying tympanic membrane.

Treatment guidelines

No treatment is necessary since over time the crust is detached from the surface of the tympanic membrane by the normal centrifugal migration of the underlying epithelium. The detached cast is then gradually carried out of the external canal on top of the normal migrating epithelium.

SEROUS OTITIS MEDIA

Definition

Serous otitis media is characterized by the presence of a non-purulent collection of *thin, watery, clear* fluid (Fig. 8.30) in the middle ear cleft.

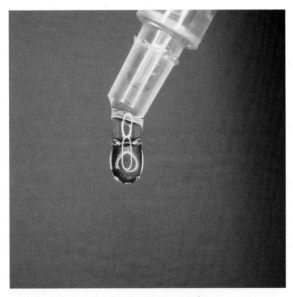

Fig. 8.30 Serous fluid. This photograph of a drop of serous fluid falling from the tip of a syringe displays the characteristic features of the fluid found in the middle ear in serous otitis media. The fluid is thin and watery in consistency, and while coloured either a yellow or golden-orange hue, the fluid is also optically transparent.

Aetiology

The basic mechanism results from a failure of the eustachian tube adequately to aerate the middle ear. The resulting chronic negative pressure within the middle ear appears to encourage an outpouring of a thin and uninfected golden-yellow watery fluid from the mucoperiosteum which lines the middle ear cleft.

Eustachian tube dysfunction can result from a variety of causes, including viral upper respiratory tract infection, enlarged adenoids, allergy of the upper respiratory tract, otitic barotrauma, cleft palate deformities, tumours of the nasopharynx, and local radiation therapy.

Symptoms

Hearing loss, ear pressure, mild earache, a stuffy or blocked feeling in the ear and clicking or popping types of tinnitus all occur.

Otoscopic appearances

The otoscopic appearances of this condition are protean and can vary from an apparently normal tympanic membrane to one which is severely retracted. When the tympanic membrane is retracted, the handle of the malleus appears to be foreshortened, chalky-white in colour and the lateral process of the malleus is unusually prominent.

The colour of the tympanic membrane will vary according to the colour of the underlying transudate. The presence of a thin serous effusion within the middle ear generally gives the tympanic membrane a yellowish (Fig. 8.31) or even an orange discoloration. Because the fluid within the middle ear is clear and transparent, the examiner can look through the fluid to see the underlying middle ear structures.

In cases of incomplete eustachian tube obstruction, air bubbles or an air–fluid level (Fig. 8.32) may be seen.

Further investigations

When there is doubt about the presence of fluid within the middle ear, or the patency of the eustachian tube is questionable, impedance audiometry or pneumatic otoscopy is often helpful in confirming the diagnosis by showing

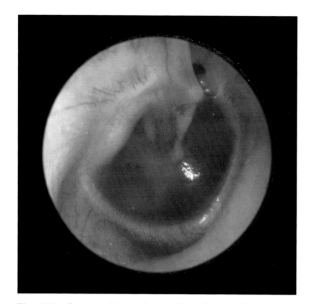

Fig. 8.31 Serous otitis media—golden effusion (right ear). The tympanic membrane is markedly retracted, the handle of the malleus is foreshortened and, as a result of the retraction, appears chalky-white in colour. The golden serous fluid present within the middle ear imparts an orange sheen to the tympanic membrane. Note how the contents of the middle ear can be clearly seen through the clear fluid.

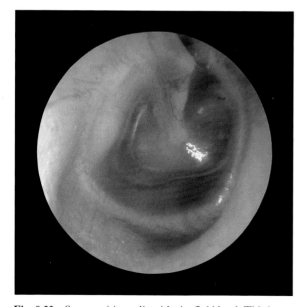

Fig. 8.32 Serous otitis media with air–fluid level. This is the same patient as shown in Figure 8.31. The patient has performed a forced Valsalva manoeuvre and pushed air up the eustachian tube and into the middle ear, displacing some of the fluid down the eustachian tube. The air–fluid level is clearly seen.

decreased mobility of the tympanic membrane and the presence of significant negative intratympanic pressure. In adults and co-operative children, tuning fork tests will reveal a conductive hearing loss. A pure tone audiogram will establish the degree of hearing impairment present.

The presence of a persistent or recurrent serous otitis media in an adult may signify the presence of an underlying carcinoma of the nasopharynx. The nasopharynx must be examined, preferably with a nasal endoscope or flexible nasopharyngoscope. If there is any doubt about the diagnosis, the nasopharynx should be examined directly under general anaesthesia to rule out the presence of an underlying carcinoma.

Therapeutic guidelines

The aim of treatment is to drain the fluid from the middle ear and to restore normal middle ear ventilation. This can be accomplished either medically or surgically.

Medical treatment is directed towards the restoration of normal eustachian tube function by the use of topical and/or systemic nasal decongestants combined with attempts at reinflation of the middle ear by the Valsalva manoeuvre (autoinflation). If medical treatment is unsuccessful, aeration of the middle ear can be achieved artificially by performing a myringotomy, aspirating the fluid and, if necessary, inserting an artificial ventilation tube (tympanostomy tube, grommet, artificial eustachian tube).

MUCOID OTITIS MEDIA (SECRETORY OTITIS MEDIA, GLUE EAR, MIDDLE EAR CATARRH)

Definition

Mucoid otitis media is characterized by the accumulation of a *thick, opalescent, tenacious,* (sticky) *mucoid* (Fig. 8.33) effusion within the middle ear cleft.

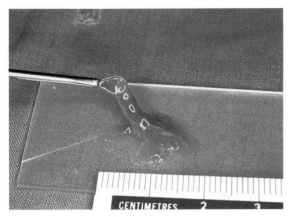

Fig. 8.33   Middle ear glue (mucoid otitis media). The characteristic tenacity of the thick mucoid effusion aspirated from a child with mucoid otitis media is illustrated in this photograph.

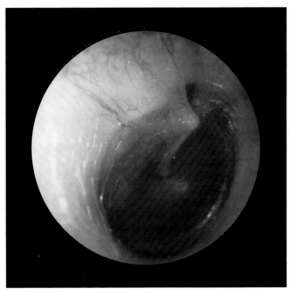

Fig. 8.34   Mucoid otitis media (right ear). Thick serous otitis media (glue ear). In this patient the tympanic membrane shows a pearly opalescent colour, due to the presence of the thick glue-like mucoid effusion fluid within the middle ear. The opalescent nature of the mucoid fluid obscures the deeper middle ear structures.

Aetiology

Mucoid otitis media is the commonest cause of acquired conductive hearing loss in children. The thick mucoid effusion which is the hallmark of mucoid otitis media is the result of the normal response of the middle ear mucosa to inflammation within the middle ear. The ascent of a viral upper respiratory infection into the middle ear via the eustachian tube is the most common cause of middle ear inflammation in childhood. Antibiotic-suppressed and incompletely resolved acute suppurative otitis media may also be a significant factor in the pathogenesis of this condition in some children.

Symptoms

The only symptom of significance in the condition is a conductive hearing loss. It should however be emphasized that this condition is frequently asymptomatic in children and may only present indirectly in the form of inattention, slow language development or poor school performance, of which it is a major cause.

Otoscopic appearances

The otoscopic appearances of mucoid otitis media are protean, and can vary from an apparently normal tympanic membrane to one which is retracted or even slightly bulging. The presence of the thick mucoid effusion within the middle ear is responsible for the dull texture and pearly-grey discoloration of the tympanic membrane (Fig. 8.34). The opalescence of the effusion usually prevents the examiner from looking through the middle ear and consequently the underlying normal middle ear structures cannot be seen. The radial vessels of the drum are often dilated (Fig. 8.35), especially when there has been a prior episode of acute suppurative otitis media. In these cases, retraction may not be present and the tympanic membrane may show flattening or even bulging. Air–fluid levels are not commonly seen in patients with mucoid otitis media.

Further investigations

Since mucoid otitis media is often asymptomatic in children, school screening programmes employing hearing tests and impedance audiometry are of great value for the early detection of this condition. A single abnormal tympanogram should not be considered an indication for referral, since many cases of eustachian tube dysfunction or serous otitis media occur transiently during the winter

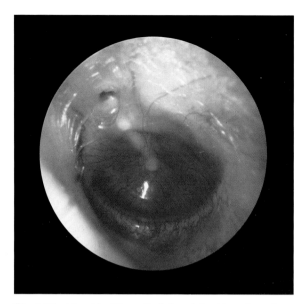

Fig. 8.35 Mucoid otitis media (left ear). In this patient, the radial vessels of the tympanic membrane are dilated (probably the result of a previous otitis media). As in Figure 8.34, the turbidity of the mucoid fluid within the middle ear prevents the long process of the incus from being seen.

months. The decision to refer a child for medical or surgical treatment should be delayed until the persistence of fluid in the middle ear has been confirmed by a second examination.

Regular otoscopic examination and audiometric testing should be performed to monitor the presence of the middle ear effusion and the degree of hearing loss. This is also indicated whenever a child presents with poor language development.

Treatment guidelines

As with serous otitis media, the aim of treatment is to drain the fluid from the middle ear and to restore normal middle ear ventilation. The best medical treatment is *tincture of time* as most middle ear effusions will resolve spontaneously over 1–2 months. If the effusion has not disappeared within this timeframe, then the fluid should be removed by performing a myringotomy and aspiration of the fluid, and the middle ear re-aerated by the insertion of an artificial ventilation tube. In some centres, adenoidectomy is also performed in an effort to improve tubal function.

MIDDLE EAR ATELECTASIS

Definition
Partial or complete severe retraction of the tympanic membrane, resulting from chronic eustachian tube dysfunction and persistent negative intratympanic pressure. Middle ear atelectasis must be differentiated from adhesive otitis media (see below).

Symptoms
These are variable; the patient may be asymptomatic or may complain of hearing loss.

Otoscopic appearances
After prolonged retraction, the tympanic membrane usually becomes thin and atrophic—presumably the result of dissolution of the fibrous middle layer (Fig. 8.36).

The thinning of the tympanic membrane allows the middle ear contents to be seen more clearly than normal and in some cases the

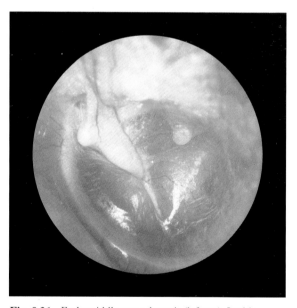

Fig. 8.36 Early middle ear atelectasis (left ear). In this patient the tympanic membrane is retracted and slightly thinned. The handle of the malleus is foreshortened and chalky-white in appearance. The long process of the incus has been destroyed by prior disease and is represented by a fibrous band. The membrane is adherent to the lenticular process of the incus and is draped over the stapedius tendon. The tympanic membrane is also plastered on to the promontory.

tympanic membrane may have become so thin that it resembles an open perforation. The use of the pneumatic attachment to the otoscope confirms the diagnosis by mobilizing the thin tympanic membrane and enables the examiner to distinguish confidently a severely retracted atrophic tympanic membrane from a large central perforation.

In less severe cases the retraction may be confined to one quadrant (Fig. 8.37), whereas in advanced cases the tympanic membrane is often firmly retracted, draped over the incus or stapes (Fig. 8.38), or even draped over the promontory.

Further investigations

Tuning fork tests and pure tone audiometry will determine the amount and nature of any hearing loss, and impedance testing will reveal the presence of negative middle ear pressure. The nose and nasopharynx must be carefully examined to exclude a treatable cause of the underlying eustachian tube dysfunction.

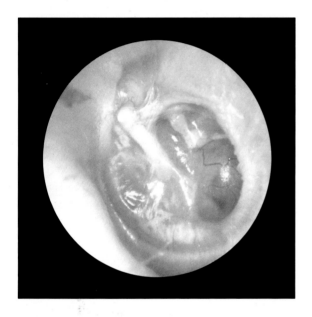

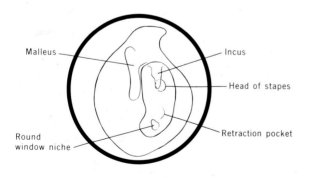

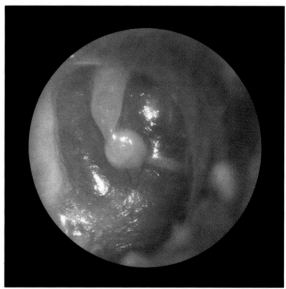

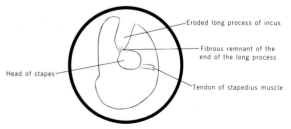

Fig. 8.37 Middle ear atelectasis—severe (left ear). In this patient the tympanic membrane has become retracted posteriorly and is draped over the incudostapedial joint. The long process of the incus is partially eroded and the posterior segment of the tympanic membrane thinned, probably representing an old healed perforation.

Fig. 8.38 Middle ear atelectasis with ossicular erosion (higher power). This is the same patient as shown in Figure 8.37 several years later. Notice the erosion of the end of the long process of the incus which is attached to the head of the stapes only by a small fibrous remnant.

Therapeutic guidelines

An effort should be made to re-aerate the middle ear. The insertion of an artificial eustachian tube into a thin atrophic tympanic membrane can be extremely difficult, especially when the drum is adherent to the promontory. A correctly placed artificial eustachian tube can be expected to re-aerate at least part of the middle ear, allowing the tympanic membrane to lift off the promontory. Since the tube will ultimately extrude, this treatment is generally of temporary value only.

RETRACTION POCKETS

Definition

A severe retraction of a segment of the tympanic membrane which produces a deep invagination (pocket).

Aetiology

Prolonged negative pressure within the middle ear may 'suck' a portion of the tympanic membrane medially. If the fibrous middle layer of the tympanic membrane has become thinned (atrophic) then a deeply invaginated pocket will form.

Symptoms

Retraction pockets are usually asymptomatic.

Otoscopic appearances

Retraction pockets form most commonly in the posterosuperior quadrant of the pars tensa (Fig. 8.39). The examiner should check that the pocket is lined with normal thin and healthy epithelium. If the patient can perform a Valsalva manoeuvre, the pocket may be seen to balloon outwards (Fig. 8.40).

Further investigations

Retraction pockets should be carefully examined to ensure that the pocket is self-cleansing. Those pockets which are unable to clean themselves may over time fill up with keratin debris and slowly enlarge until they form a cholesteatoma.

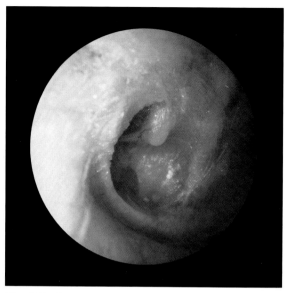

Fig. 8.39 Posterior retraction pocket (right ear). The posterior portion of the tympanic membrane has been sucked medially producing a retraction pocket. Note how the posterior portion of the retraction pocket extends deep to the bony annulus.

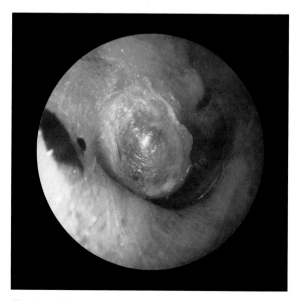

Fig. 8.40 Retraction pocket post-autoinflation (right ear). Following autoinflation (Valsalva manoeuvre) the sudden inflow of air into the middle ear has blown the retraction pocket laterally into the external canal.

Treatment guidelines

Careful follow-up as mentioned above is important to prevent the development of a cholesteatoma.

ADHESIVE OTITIS MEDIA

Definition

A long-standing process in which the tympanic membrane is retracted medially and *permanently tethered* to the medial wall of the middle ear by fibrous adhesions which have developed in the middle ear as the result of previous inflammatory middle ear disease.

Aetiology

These fibrous adhesions may arise as a complication of any inflammatory process, whether suppurative or non-suppurative otitis media, which has been severe enough to damage the mucosal lining of the middle ear. During healing, fibrous adhesions (which represent scar formation) may develop. In mild cases, only a few adhesions may be present while in the more severely affected ear these adhesions are more numerous and ankylosis of the ossicular chain can occur.

Symptoms

The principal complaint is hearing loss and there is often a history of previous episodes of otitis media, especially in childhood.

Otoscopic appearances

The key otoscopic feature of adhesive otitis media is severe and irreversible retraction of the tympanic membrane (Fig. 8.41.). The appearance of the tympanic membrane may vary from minimal scarring to overall thickening and opacity. Changes of severe retraction, atrophic areas or tympanosclerotic plaques may also be present. Pneumatic otoscopy almost always discloses severe impairment or even a total absence of tympanic membrane mobility.

Further investigations

Impedance testing will show severely diminished

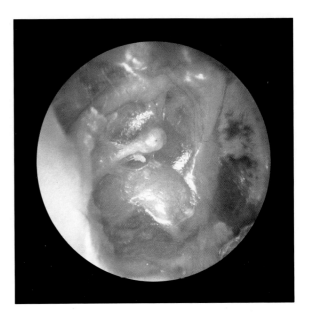

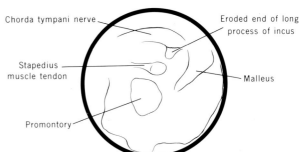

Fig. 8.41 Adhesive otitis media (right ear). In this patient the tympanic membrane has become retracted, thinned and adherent to the medial wall of the middle ear. The tympanic membrane is plastered over the promontory. The stapedius muscle tendon and head of the stapes are clearly visible and the long process of the incus is eroded and no longer in contact with the head of the stapes. There is also seen severe retraction in the posterosuperior quadrant, with the chorda tympani nerve being visible. There is tympanosclerosis anteriorly and the shadow of the round window niche is also visible.

or even absent middle ear mobility and pure tone audiometry will measure the degree of conductive hearing loss present.

Therapeutic guidelines

Surgical treatment of advanced cases of adhesive otitis media is unrewarding, especially when abnormal eustachian tube function coexists. A hearing aid is of use in cases of severe ossicular fixation and severe hearing loss. The primary aim should be to prevent the formation of fibrous adhesions from episodes of suppurative ear disease or recurrent serous otitis media in early life. Middle ear infections should be treated with full courses of appropriate antibiotics and chronic serous effusions drained.

TYMPANOSCLEROSIS (CHALK PATCHES)

Definition
The deposition of plaques of hyalinized collagen beneath the lining epithelium of the middle ear.

Aetiology
Tympanosclerotic plaques appear to result from the organization of both fibrinous exudates and granulation tissue after previous severe acute otitis media.

Symptoms
There may be no symptoms, as small patches of tympanosclerosis situated in the tympanic membrane do not appear to interfere with normal function. There is often a history of previous otitis media in childhood and particularly of ventilating tube insertion, which may stimulate this reaction. Tympanosclerotic plaques occur very commonly in the tympanic membrane and in this location rarely produce symptoms. Tympanosclerosis involving the middle ear mucosa and ossicles is rare; however, when middle ear tympanosclerosis occurs it is usually associated with a conductive hearing loss and unfortunately this type of tympanosclerosis is very difficult to manage surgically.

Otoscopic appearances
Tympanosclerotic plaques confined to the tympanic membrane always occur in the pars tensa and may vary in size from small, chalky-white patches (Fig. 8.42) to large plaques involving the entire tympanic membrane (Fig. 8.43). In rare cases the tympanosclerotic deposits

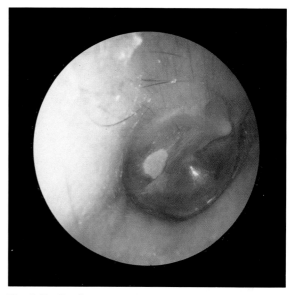

Fig. 8.42   Small tympanosclerotic plaque (right ear). There is a small discrete round white plaque of tympanosclerosis visible in the posterior quadrant of the tympanic membrane. This is of no clinical significance.

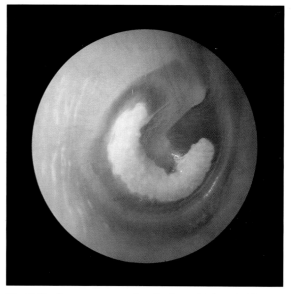

Fig. 8.43   Large tympanosclerotic plaque (right ear). Note the large crescent-shaped plaque of tympanosclerosis. Of no significance by itself, tympanosclerosis of the membrane always signifies previous ear disease.

may envelope the ossicles (Fig. 8.44) causing partial or total fixation of the ossicular chain.

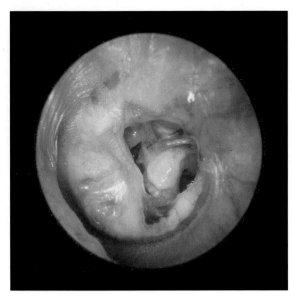

Fig. 8.44   Heavy tympanosclerosis (left ear). In this patient the tympanic membrane is diffusely involved with tympanosclerosis. There is also a large tympanosclerotic deposit visible in the middle ear, seen through the posterior perforation.

CHRONIC SUPPURATIVE OTITIS MEDIA

Definition

Chronic suppurative otitis media (CSOM) is a disorder of the middle ear cleft, characterized by hearing loss and persistent or recurrent discharge. This state of affairs occurs when an acute inflammation produces irreversible changes affecting the structure and function of the middle ear cleft. For clinical purposes, CSOM is considered to be *safe* or *unsafe* depending upon the location and the type of pathological process within the middle ear. When the lining membrane involved is respiratory in type (derived from the tubo-tympanic recess; Fig. 8.45), recurrent otorrhoea and hearing loss may be troublesome but there is generally no great danger to the patient.

Further investigations

Tympanosclerotic plaques confined to the tympanic membrane do not cause hearing loss. In extensive cases, with involvement of the middle ear and ossicles, audiometric testing will indicate the presence of a conductive hearing loss due to interference with ossicular chain mobility. Tympanometry will usually indicate the presence of normal middle ear pressure and decreased tympanic membrane mobility. The ear should be examined with the operating microscope to establish the extent of the disease and to differentiate tympanosclerosis from a coexisting cholesteatoma.

Therapeutic guidelines

The aim of the treatment is to alleviate any hearing loss present. This is usually accomplished by the use of amplification (a hearing aid), since surgical reconstruction is usually unrewarding.

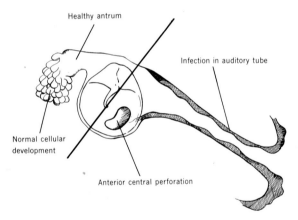

Fig. 8.45   The features of the *safe* ear. (After H. Ludman.)

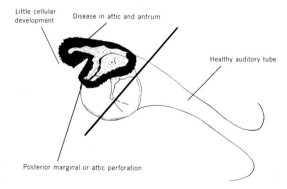

Fig. 8.46   The features of the *unsafe* ear. (After H. Ludman.)

If, however, the squamous epithelium in the area of the attic and mastoid antrum (posterosuperiorly; Fig. 8.46) becomes diseased, erosion of the underlying bone is likely to occur and serious complications can follow. In unsafe CSOM, an enlarging pocket of squamous epithelium derived from Shrapnell's membrane can be invaginated into the attic of the middle ear to form a cholesteatoma which slowly erodes the adjacent ossicles and bony walls of the middle ear and mastoid.

Symptoms

The symptoms of CSOM are variable, consisting primarily of hearing loss and recurrent painless otorrhoea. If complications develop, the patient may present with facial paralysis, vertigo, pain and the symptoms and signs of meningitis or other intracranial pathology.

Otoscopic appearances

The otoscopic appearances of CSOM are variable. In tubotympanic disease, a central perforation is usually seen. In atticoantral disease, a marginal perforation, an attic perforation, an attic crust or a frank cholesteatoma may be encountered.

CENTRAL PERFORATION

Definition

A perforation in the pars tensa of the tympanic membrane which does not extend to involve the annulus is termed a central perforation. These perforations are designated as *safe*, since they are usually not associated with cholesteatoma or with the intracranial spread of infection.

Aetiology

Most central perforations result from a previous acute otitis media and represent a failure in the healing of a tympanic membrane perforation. Central perforations may also follow severe trauma.

Symptoms

Even a large perforation may be asymptomatic and only detected during a routine medical examination. Most patients, however, are aware of hearing loss and complain of intermittent discharge following upper respiratory tract infections or after the entry of water into the ear.

Otoscopic appearances

Central perforations may vary in size from a small pinhole (Fig. 8.47), to a virtually total kidney-shaped perforation (Fig. 8.48). Some middle ear structures can often be partly seen through a large subtotal perforation. The middle ear may be perfectly dry and the mucoperiosteal lining healthy in appearance. If the middle ear is infected, mucopurulent material (Fig. 8.49) will be seen through the perforation and the mucosa is usually red and oedematous (Fig. 8.50).

In severely infected cases, mucopus, which may vary in colour and consistency, drains outwards through the perforation and can fill the external canal. In an acutely inflamed ear the discharge may be pulsatile.

When a large perforation heals, the fibrous middle layer of the pars tensa is deficient, so that a thin semi-transparent membrane resembling an open perforation will be seen (Fig. 8.51). Gentle use of the pneumatic attachment to the otoscope

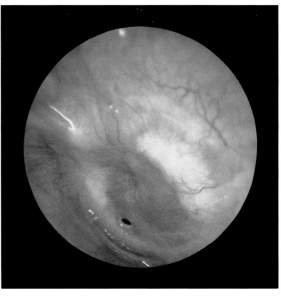

Fig. 8.47 Pinhole perforation (left ear). There is a small pinhole perforation in the anteroinferior quadrant. Note also the dense tympanosclerosis posteriorly.

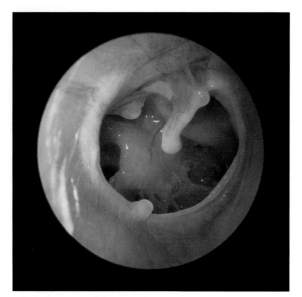

Fig. 8.48 Total perforation (right ear). There is a total perforation, through which the long process of the incus and its articulation with the head of the stapes and the stapedius tendon can be seen posterosuperiorly. The round window niche is also visible in the posteroinferior quadrant. There is excessive mucus in the middle ear and an abnormal thickening of the mucosa.

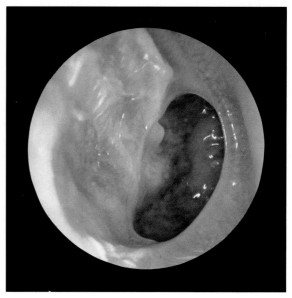

Fig. 8.50 Central perforation with infected middle ear mucosa (right ear). Notice the erythema and oedema of the middle ear mucosa which can be seen through this rather large anterior perforation. The posterior edge of the perforation is adherent to the promontory.

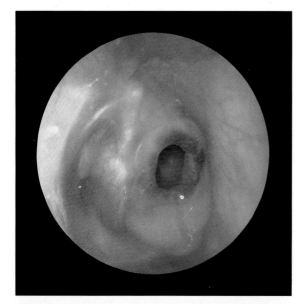

Fig. 8.49 Infected central perforation (right ear). In this patient the middle ear is chronically infected. The central perforation is surrounded by a ring of granulation tissue and yellowish mucopurulent exudate can be seen draining into the external canal.

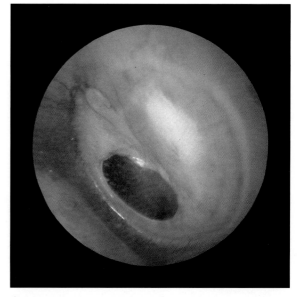

Fig. 8.51 Healed perforation (left ear). The anteroinferior perforation in this patient has healed with a thin semi-transparent membrane.

will, however, demonstrate that the tympanic membrane is intact.

Further investigations

If the ear is infected, a swab should be taken for culture studies. An audiogram is necessary to assess the degree of hearing loss.

Therapeutic guidelines

The patient should be instructed to keep water out of the ear in order to avoid repeated middle ear infections. Small perforations will often heal spontaneously, whereas tympanoplastic surgery to close a persistent perforation may be indicated in those patients with troublesome hearing loss or recurrent otorrhoea after swimming. Because the thinned segment of a healed perforation lacks the strength of a normal drum, forceful syringing may result in re-perforation.

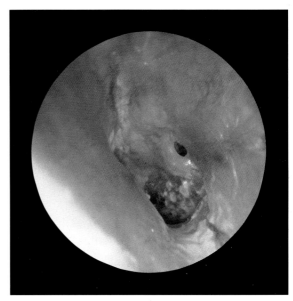

Fig. 8.52 Small marginal perforation (left ear). There is a small pinpoint marginal perforation in the annulus posterosuperiorly. This type of marginal perforation is considered unsafe since there may be an underlying cholesteatoma.

MARGINAL PERFORATION

Definition

A marginal perforation is one which involves the annulus of the pars tensa of the tympanic membrane. These perforations are considered *unsafe*, since they are frequently associated with cholesteatoma.

Symptoms

The symptoms are essentially the same as those for central perforations.

Aetiology

Previous middle ear infections and long-standing eustachian tube dysfunction.

Otoscopic appearances

Marginal perforations involve the annulus, and vary in size from a small defect (Fig. 8.52) to a large subtotal perforation of the tympanic membrane (Fig. 8.53). A marginal perforation located in the posterosuperior quadrant of the tympanic membrane is especially worrisome, since this is most likely to be associated with an underlying cholesteatoma.

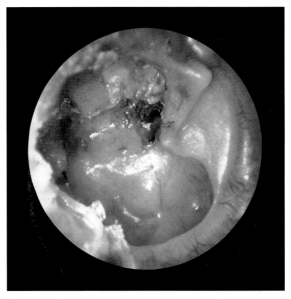

Fig. 8.53 Marginal perforation (right ear). In this patient there is a large posterosuperior perforation containing keratin debris. There has been gross erosion of bone and healing on to the floor of the middle ear of a thin neomembrane. The posterosuperior marginal perforation with erosion of the canal wall represents a cholesteatoma.

Further investigations

These should include audiometric testing, culture of any discharge present, a thorough examination of the ear with the operating microscope, and if there is any evidence of bone erosion from an underlying cholesteatoma, appropriate mastoid X-rays or a high-resolution computerized tomography scan should be requested.

Therapeutic guidelines

Obvious infection is treated as described previously, but the examiner must always have a high index of suspicion about a cholesteatoma either being present or developing within the middle ear cleft. Careful follow-up of these patients by a specialist is advisable.

ATTIC CRUSTS

The presence of a crust (Fig. 8.54) or piece of wax obscuring the posterosuperior part of Shrapnell's membrane must never be dismissed as trivial, since an underlying perforation or even a cholesteatoma is probably present. Using the operating microscope it is generally possible to remove attic crusts using instruments and suction.

If a small retraction pocket of an intact pars tensa is discovered, no further treatment is required immediately and the patient can be carefully followed. If, however, the perforation contains an obvious collection of whitish keratin squames (Fig. 8.55), the presence of a cholesteatoma hidden within the middle ear is highly likely and further treatment including a mastoid exploration should be considered.

ATTIC PERFORATION

An attic perforation (Fig. 8.56) is the hallmark of unsafe, chronic suppurative otitis media. After treating overt infection with aural toilet, suction and local antibiotic drugs, an examination of the ear with the operating microscope is necessary to determine whether granulation tissue or a cholesteatoma lies within. Extensive underlying bony destruction of the incus and medial wall of the attic may have occurred 'around the corner' out of view and cannot be identified through a

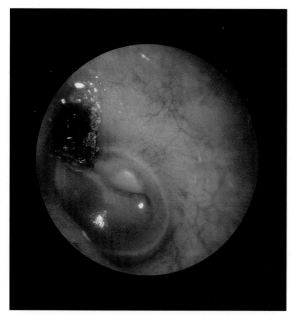

Fig. 8.54 Attic crust (left ear). This patient presented with a waxy crust overlying the posterosuperior quadrant.

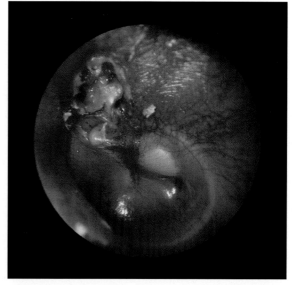

Fig. 8.55 Attic perforation. After the removal of the crust shown in Figure 8.54, an attic perforation was visible. The white keratin debris seen within the perforation is characteristic of a cholesteatoma.

small attic perforation. Examination of the ear under general anaesthesia will be necessary and if doubt remains about the presence of active disease within, a surgical exploration of the ear is then required.

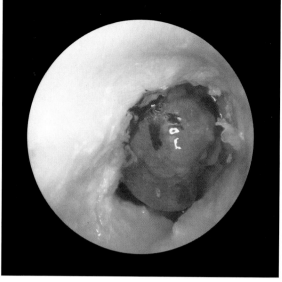

Fig. 8.57 Inflammatory aural polyp (right ear). In this patient a pale pink fleshy polyp was visible at the entrance of the external meatus.

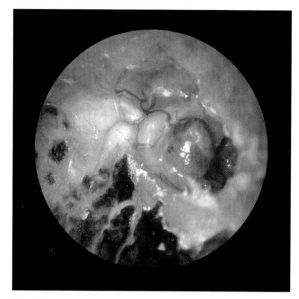

Fig. 8.56 Attic granulation tissue. Under higher magnification, the presence of a granulation tissue polyp within the attic perforation is clearly visible and indicates a high probability of an underlying cholesteatoma.

AURAL POLYP

A polyp in the external ear may arise either from the external auditory canal or from the middle ear. Aural polyps are usually inflammatory in origin and occur as the result of chronic suppurative otitis media (Figs 8.57 and 8.58). Occasionally, a neoplasm will present as an aural polyp. Injudicious manipulation of an inflammatory aural polyp may result in troublesome bleeding. When an aural polyp is discovered, the patient should be promptly referred to an otologist, who will remove it in the operating theatre under general anaesthesia.

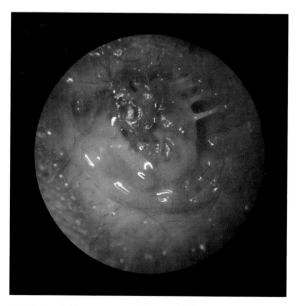

Fig. 8.58 Inflammatory aural polyp (right ear). A fleshy pink inflammatory aural polyp is seen within the external meatus surrounded by creamy-white mucopurulent exudate.

CHOLESTEATOMA

Definition

A cholesteatoma is a cystic collection of keratin debris, produced and enclosed by a sac of stratified squamous keratinizing epithelium located within the middle ear cleft.

Aetiology

The precise mechanism of cholesteatoma formation is unclear, but in most cases it is likely that chronic eustachian tube obstruction leads to prolonged negative intratympanic pressure, which draws a pocket of the stratified squamous epithelium lining the outer aspect of the posterosuperior segment of the pars flaccida or pars tensa into the middle ear space. The keratin desquamated from the epithelium lining this pocket collects within, producing a gradually enlarging cyst. As the cyst expands it erodes the surrounding bony walls of the middle ear and ossicles.

Otoscopic appearances

In advanced cases, a cholesteatoma will present as an exuberant, greasy, whitish mass of keratin squames (Figs 8.59, 8.60), protruding through a perforation in the posterior portion of the pars flaccida or under the posterior malleolar fold. More commonly, the only sign of a large cholesteatoma in the mastoid antrum or air cells may be a few shiny white keratin squames visible through a small attic perforation (Fig. 8.55). It is dangerous to overlook the presence of active squamous epithelium located deep to the tympanic membrane or in the mastoid air cells, since over a period of time gradual bony erosion may lead to life-threatening complications such as labyrinthitis, meningitis or brain abscess.

Further investigations

It is crucial to assess the extent of the disease. Although an examination of the ear under the operating microscope either in the clinic or under a general anaesthetic may reveal the presence of a cholesteatoma, it is impossible to estimate the extent of inward and backward spread by otoscopy or microscopy alone. Mastoid X-rays

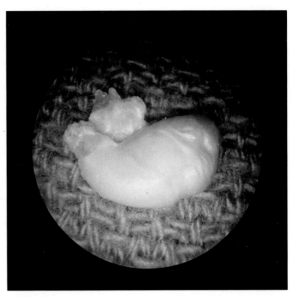

Fig. 8.59 Cholesteatoma debris. This pearly-white plug of keratin debris was removed from the mouth of an attic cholesteatoma.

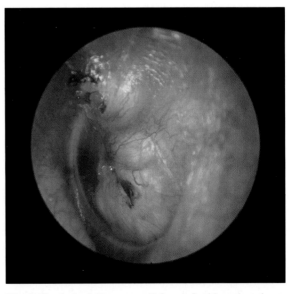

Fig. 8.60 Attic cholesteatoma (left ear). In this patient the attic crust heralds the presence of a cholesteatoma. Note the whitish cholesteatoma sac which can be seen behind the intact tympanic membrane.

and especially a computerized tomography (CT) scan are helpful in demonstrating the extent of bony erosion.

Therapeutic guidelines

Small cholesteatomas which can be completely cleaned by suction under the operating microscope may be managed by regular debridement and close observation. With larger pockets, in all but the elderly, the treatment of this disease is surgical (Fig. 8.61) and requires a mastoid exploration with either removal or exteriorization of the cholesteatoma.

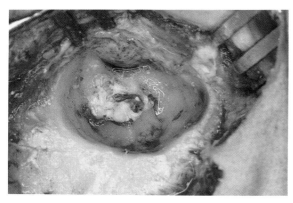

Fig. 8.61   Cholesteatoma eroding into the mastoid. At operation, a large cholesteatoma (skin-lined sac) was found eroding posteriorly into the bony mastoid process.

GLOMUS TUMOURS OF THE MIDDLE EAR (SYNONYMS: CHEMODECTOMA, GLOMUS JUGULARE, GLOMUS TYMPANICUM)

Definition

A slowly growing, locally invasive, vascular tumour arising from chemoreceptor tissue (glomus bodies), which are quite widely distributed in the head and neck. They are particularly prevalent in the tissue around the jugular bulb (glomus jugulare), and on the promontory of the middle ear (glomus tympanicum). These tumours occur five times more commonly in females than in males.

Symptoms

The glomus tympanicum will usually present with a unilateral hearing loss and an associated pulsatile roaring or rushing tinnitus. A glomus jugulare tumour may, in addition, present as a bleeding polyp in the ear canal. Cranial nerve

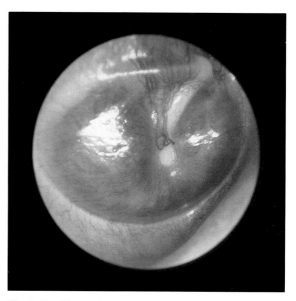

Fig. 8.62   Glomus jugulare tumour (right ear). The glomus tumour in this patient is seen as a bright red mass filling the middle ear and pushing the tympanic membrane laterally.

involvement is common, particularly facial and vagal palsy.

Otoscopic examination

The earliest sign is a redness behind the tympanic membrane which is caused by the presence of this highly vascular tumour within the middle ear. The tumour may appear as a blue or red 'rising sun', seen behind the inferior portion of the tympanic membrane. The red colour of the tympanic membrane often decreases if it can be 'lifted off' the tumour by the pneumatic otoscope. In more advanced cases, the tumour may present as a red vascular polyp (Fig. 8.62) within the external canal, which can bleed profusely on manipulation.

Further investigations

A careful examination of cranial nerves VII, IX, X, XI and XII must be performed to determine whether extratympanic spread and involvement of the jugular foramen has occurred. A pulsatile systolic bruit may be heard over the mastoid. If the tympanometer is used at its most sensitive setting, pulsatile movements transmitted from the vascular tumour to the tympanic membrane may be recorded.

A jugular venogram will demonstrate the relationship of this lesion to the jugular bulb and a carotid arteriogram will help both in demonstrating the vascular nature of the lesion as well as determining its blood supply. A CT scan may also be used to assist in delineating the extent of the tumour.

Therapeutic guidelines

In all patients with unilateral pulsatile tinnitus, the possibility of an underlying vascular tumour or arteriovenous malformation should be considered.

An abnormally high jugular bulb (Fig. 8.64) may also give a 'rising sun' appearance similar to that of a glomus jugulare tumour.

The treatment of glomus tumours may be by radiotherapy, embolization of the feeding arterial blood supply, surgical extirpation or a combination thereof.

SQUAMOUS CELL CARCINOMA (SYNONYM: EPITHELIOMA)

Definition

A rare malignant tumour arising from the skin of the external auditory canal or the lining of the tympanic cavity (Fig. 8.65).

Aetiology

The exact aetiology is unknown; however, there is strong circumstantial evidence that chronic irritation from prolonged otorrhoea is a significant aetiological factor. These tumours occur most commonly between the fourth and sixth decades of life.

Symptoms

Pain in the presence of chronic otorrhoea is the most common symptom. The development of

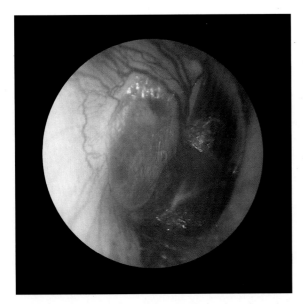

Fig. 8.63 Glomus tumour (right ear). Notice the red vascular friable glomus tumour filling the anteroinferior quadrant and displacing the tympanic membrane outwards.

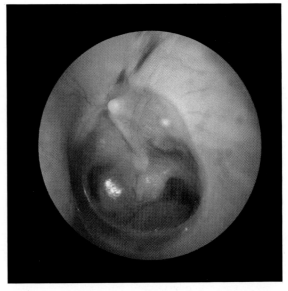

Fig. 8.64 The blue mass seen in the inferior quadrant of the tympanic membrane is an abnormally high jugular bulb.

pain in any chronically infected ear should be considered a warning sign that a malignant tumour may be present. An exuberant polyp or growth extending into the meatus, especially those which are nodular, friable and haemorrhagic, is also a warning signal. The definitive diagnosis is made by histological examination of a biopsy specimen.

In advanced cases there may be evidence of associated cranial nerve paralysis, particularly of the VIIth nerve.

Otoscopic appearance

The presence of an aural polyp or growth showing a nodular or friable appearance is frequently encountered.

Further investigations

These patients should be promptly referred for a specialist opinion and treatment.

Treatment guidelines

If practical, treatment usually involves wide surgical excision combined with radiotherapy. Radiotherapy alone is frequently utilized in those lesions which cannot be completely excised, or in the event of recurrence.

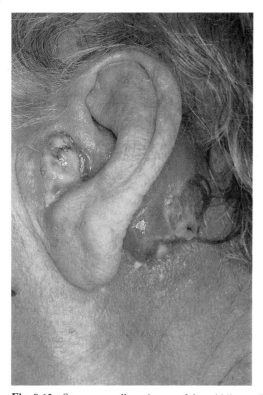

Fig. 8.65 Squamous cell carcinoma of the middle ear. The external auditory canal is narrowed by a fleshy mass which has eroded posteriorly and can be seen ulcerating through the mastoid process.

9. Postoperative appearances

MYRINGOTOMY

Definition

A surgical incision through the tympanic membrane.

Indications

Myringotomies are usually performed for one of three reasons: to determine if fluid is present in the middle ear, to establish drainage of the purulent contents of the middle ear in the advanced stages of acute suppurative otitis media and to aspirate non-purulent effusions.

The anteroinferior quadrant of the tympanic membrane provides the safest location for a myringotomy incision because in this area there is little risk of damage to the ossicular chain. A myringotomy incision should never be performed in the posterosuperior quadrant because of the high risk in this area of damaging the long process of the incus and the stapes.

In untreated acute otitis media, the presence of pus under pressure in the middle ear eventually produces a marked outward bulge of the inferior quadrant of the tympanic membrane. In such cases, a timely myringotomy in the most bulging portion of the tympanic membrane will often relieve the patient's pain by decompressing the tympanic membrane and allowing pus to drain from the middle ear. There is considerable controversy about the actual benefit of this type of 'hot myringotomy', and today acute otitis media is not commonly considered as a strong indication for a myringotomy.

When a myringotomy is necessary for the aspiration of fluid from a non-infected middle ear, e.g. in serous or mucoid otitis media, a radial incision is preferred, since fewer of the radial tympanic blood vessels are transected (Fig. 9.1).

In acute suppurative otitis media, a circumferential incision has traditionally been recommended to promote freer drainage (Fig. 9.2). In practice, in these patients, a circumferential incision causes little additional bleeding, since ischaemia of the tympanic capillaries is usually present by this stage.

Spontaneous closure of the myringotomy incision will usually occur within 5–7 days after

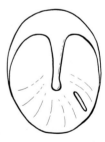

Fig. 9.1 Anteroinferior radial myringotomy for serous otitis media (right ear).

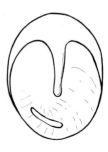

Fig. 9.2 Wide circumferential myringotomy for acute otitis media (right ear).

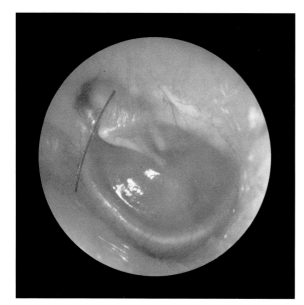

Fig. 9.3 Serous otitis media. The tympanic membrane is retracted and the handle of the malleus fore-shortened. The middle ear is filled with a clear golden-yellow serous fluid which gives the tympanic membrane a yellow discoloration (left ear).

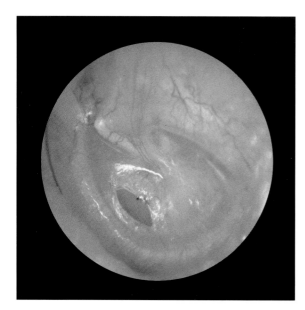

Fig. 9.4 Serous otitis media, post myringotomy. This is the same patient as illustrated in Figure 9.3. The fluid has been aspirated through a small circumferential myringotomy (left ear). Notice how the yellow discoloration of the tympanic membrane has disappeared.

drainage from the middle ear ceases, leaving a barely perceptible scar.

Currently, myringotomies are most commonly performed in the treatment of serous otitis media (Figs 9.3 and 9.4) which has not resolved after conservative measures. In children a general anaesthetic is preferred, while in adults local anaesthesia may be obtained by infiltrating lignocaine into the skin of the posterior canal wall or by means of an iontophoretic technique. In the adult, topical anaesthesia may also be produced by applying a drop of 10% phenol solution by means of a Derlacki applicator to the area where the myringotomy incision is to be made. The phenol blanches the anaesthetized area of the tympanic membrane epithelium, and an incision can be easily and painlessly made in this whitened area. With this technique, anaesthesia is obtained in approximately 15 seconds.

Recent studies in Europe have shown that if a eutectic mixture of local anaesthetics is applied to the surface of the tympanic membrane in the form of a cream (Emla cream; Astra Pharmaceuticals), excellent topical anaesthesia of the tympanic membrane is produced within 10–15 minutes of application. It should be noted that many adults are capable of tolerating a myringotomy without any anaesthesia, providing that a sharp myringotome is used.

TYMPANOSTOMY TUBES (SYNONYMS: ARTIFICIAL EUSTACHIAN TUBES, GROMMETS, DRAINS, BOBBINS, PRESSURE EQUALIZING TUBES, VENTILATION TUBES)

The commonest surgical procedure currently performed in children in the USA is the insertion of an artificial eustachian tube into a myringotomy incision. These tubes are currently available in a wide range of sizes, shapes, colours and materials (Figs 9.5 and 9.6) and consequently, the examiner should not be surprised to encounter an unfamiliar variety of tube. Most tubes are designed with an inner flange to delay extrusion, and often feature an outer flange to prevent the tube falling into the middle ear (Fig

9.5). The very fact that there are so many different types of ventilation tubes available indicates that none is uniformly successful.

Most cases of conductive hearing loss caused by intractable chronic serous or mucoid otitis media require prolonged artificial middle ear ventilation. Since most myringotomy incisions heal spontaneously within a few days, little time is left for eustachian tube function to recover and consequently the middle ear effusion will tend to recur. For this reason a ventilation tube is inserted through the myringotomy incision.

The primary function of the artificial eustachian tube is to provide ventilation of the middle ear cleft by allowing the free passage of air through the tympanic membrane (Figs 9.5 and 9.6). These ventilation tubes may also act as drains both for middle ear effusions and for the purulent material which may develop during a subsequent episode of otitis media (Fig. 9.7).

Because the lumen of most tubes will allow water to pass from the deep external canal into the middle ear, care should be exercised while showering, hair-washing or swimming to prevent water entering into the middle ear and the possibility of a subsequent infection.

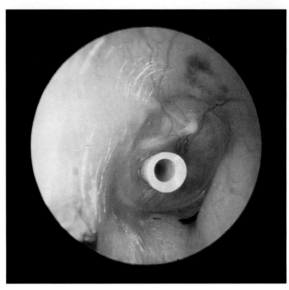

Fig. 9.6 Artificial eustachian tube (T tube). A blue silastic T tube can be seen in the centre of the tympanic membrane (right ear).

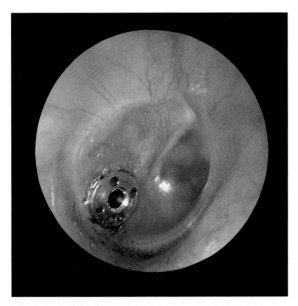

Fig. 9.5 Artificial eustachian tube (grommet). A stainless steel Reuter bobbin is in place in the tympanic membrane (right ear).

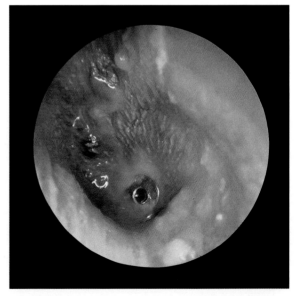

Fig. 9.7 Discharging tube. This patient has developed an acute otitis media. Creamy-white mucopurulent material is draining out of the stainless steel tube. The upper portion of the tympanic membrane is oedematous and erythematous as a result of this acute infection (left ear).

For swimming, the ear is best protected by the use of ear plugs and a bathing cap. Many commercially available ear plugs are unsuitable and do not provide the degree of protection required. Custom-moulded swim plugs, if used properly, are generally to be preferred. For bathing and showering, the use of a plug made simply of cotton-wool impregnated with petroleum jelly is satisfactory, although lambswool coated with lanolin may afford greater protection.

BLOCKED TYMPANOSTOMY TUBE

For a tympanostomy tube to function properly, its lumen must remain patent. Premature blockage of the lumen (Fig. 9.8) with inspissated mucus or serous debris may lead to an early return of the middle ear effusion; replacement of the tube may then be required, although the use of ear drops may sometimes soften the debris and clear the tube. This should be given a trial before subjecting the child to another anaesthetic.

Sometimes, ventilation tubes are repeatedly ejected after only a short time. Here the situation should be re-evaluated, and the pros and cons of a hearing aid discussed relative to the repeated anaesthetics required for tube insertion, if the primary reason for the tube is the correction of hearing loss.

EXTRUDING TYMPANOSTOMY TUBE

As a result of the normal outward movement of the epithelial cells from the surface of the tympanic membrane along the ear canal, a tympanostomy tube will normally be extruded spontaneously from the tympanic membrane 6–12 months after insertion (Fig. 9.9). The underlying myringotomy incision heals in most cases. Fortunately, tubes rarely fall medially into the middle ear.

After the tube has been extruded from the tympanic membrane, migration outwards into the superficial portion of the external auditory canal normally occurs (Figs 9.10 and 9.11). The tube, often encrusted with wax, may drop out of

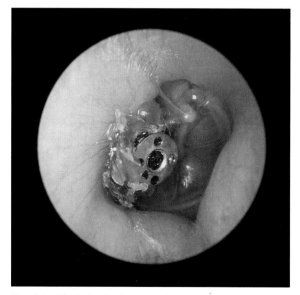

Fig. 9.8 Blocked tube. In this patient the central lumen of the tube has become blocked with a crust of desiccated serous fluid and is no longer functioning as a source of ventilation for the middle ear (left ear).

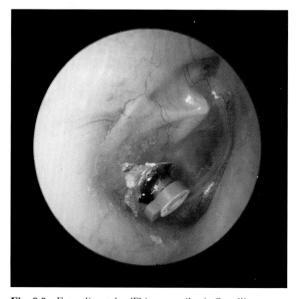

Fig. 9.9 Extruding tube. This green silastic Castelli membrane ventilation tube is being extruded from the surface of the tympanic membrane (right ear).

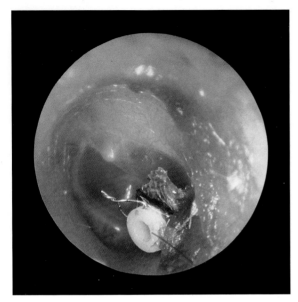

Fig. 9.10 Extruding tube. This white polyethylene tube has been extruded and is lying in some wax in the posteroinferior quadrant. This type of tube has a small wire attached to make removal easier (left ear).

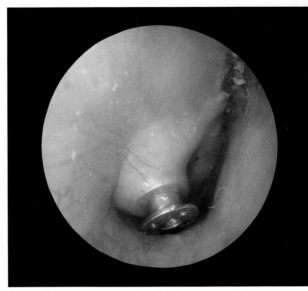

Fig. 9.12 Tube extruding secondary to infection. As the result of an episode of acute otitis media, this tube is extruding prematurely, 1 month after placement (right ear).

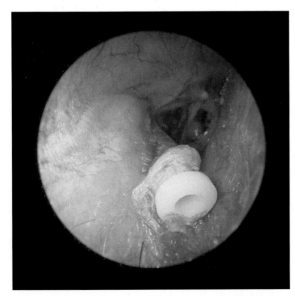

Fig. 9.11 Extruded tube. In this patient a white silastic tube has been extruded and is being carried laterally on top of the outward migrating skin of the bony canal (right ear).

the ear spontaneously or can be removed with crocodile forceps.

If the ear becomes infected, the tube may extrude more rapidly (Fig. 9.12). In many atelectatic ears, tympanostomy tubes are frequently rejected quite rapidly, possibly due to atrophic changes in the tympanic membrane. This is unfortunate because the ventilation tubes are most needed in this situation.

TYMPANOSTOMY TUBE FOREIGN BODY GRANULOMA (TUBE GRANULOMA)

In approximately 0.5% of cases, the tympanostomy tube stimulates the development of a keratin foreign body granuloma. This is characterized by the presence of granulation tissue with or without mucopurulent discharge adjacent to the tympanostomy tube (Fig. 9.13). This exuberant granulation tissue may be responsible for the development of a profuse and usually painless otorrhoea, which is frequently tinged with blood. A tube granuloma is treated by removal of the tube and the associated

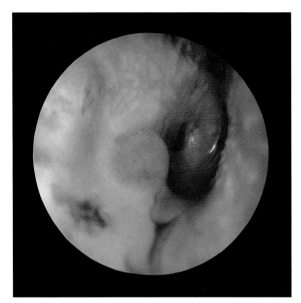

Fig. 9.13 Tube granuloma. A red mass of granulation tissue with associated surrounding mucopurulent exudate is visible in the 7 o'clock position, obscuring the tube (right ear).

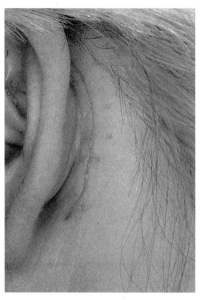

Fig. 9.14 Post-auricular scar. The post-auricular sulcus should always be examined to ascertain if a tell-tale surgical scar is present (left ear).

granulation tissue.

POST-TYMPANOPLASTY

Tympanoplasty is a generic term used to describe those surgical procedures which are performed to reconstruct the hearing mechanism of the middle ear. The term *tympanoplasty* by definition includes surgical repair of the tympanic membrane, but may also, and often does, include reconstructive surgery of the ossicular chain. More specifically, myringoplasty denotes that the tympanic membrane has been repaired or replaced and the term *ossiculoplasty* is used if a discontinuity of the ossicular chain is repaired. Tympanoplastic procedures often combine both elements as for example in cases of middle ear damage resulting from trauma or chronic infection.

The final appearance of the operated ear varies and indeed may be otoscopically normal. If a post-aural (Fig. 9. 14) or an end-aural (Fig. 9.15) incision has been used to approach the tympanic membrane or middle ear, a faint tell-tale scar will be present. It is good practice to inspect both the post-auricular skin and the sulcus between the

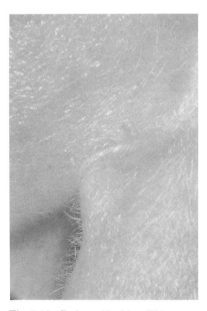

Fig. 9.15 End-aural incision. This incision leaves a characteristic scar running between the upper part of the tragus and the crus of the helix (right ear).

crus of the helix and the tragus, even if there is no clear past history of ear surgery, since an operation carried out in early childhood may have been forgotten by the patient. In contrast, an endomeatal incision (an incision in the skin of the bony external auditory canal) will usually heal without scarring and cannot be detected.

When the graft material used for a successful myringoplasty is temporalis fascia, the tympanic membrane will generally assume an almost normal appearance (Fig. 9.16). If the result is less than perfect, scarring of the tympanic membrane or fullness ('blunting') of the anterior recess may be evident. It is just occasionally possible to appreciate the results of an ossiculoplasty through a thin or retracted intact tympanic membrane, but otherwise there are usually no visible clues as to what has transpired within the middle ear.

MASTOID CAVITY

In the course of a radical or modified radical mastoidectomy operation, both the posterior bony wall of the external auditory canal and the outer attic wall are removed. This marsupializes the mastoid antrum and air cells so that the cavity produced after the surgical exenteration of disease (chronic inflammation, cholesteatoma, neoplasms) will communicate freely with the external auditory canal.

Otoscopic appearances

The external meatus should have been enlarged (*meatoplasty*) to provide proper aeration as well as easy postoperative access to the mastoid cavity for routine cleansing (Fig. 9.17). By angling the otoscope backwards and upwards the mastoid cavity can be seen. In cases where an inadequate meatoplasty has been performed and the external canal is narrow, or where the posterior canal wall (facial ridge) has been insufficiently lowered, it may be extremely difficult to obtain a satisfactory view of the cavity. In the case of a modified radical mastoidectomy performed through a post-auricular approach, failure to inspect the post-auricular skin for scarring can result in a small cavity being overlooked during a cursory examination of the ear. Figure 9.18 shows the

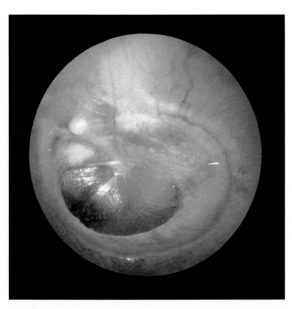

Fig. 9.16 Post-tympanoplasty. This patient had a successful tympanoplasty to close a large central perforation. The tympanic membrane is intact and the defect has been replaced by a healed thin membrane (left ear).

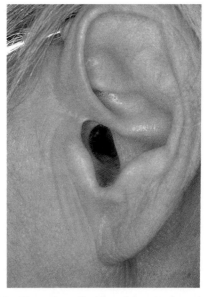

Fig. 9.17 Meatoplasty. In this patient an end-aural scar is visible just in front of the crus of the helix. Notice how the meatoplasty has widened the meatus, thereby allowing the physician ready access to the mastoid cavity for purposes of aural toilet (left ear).

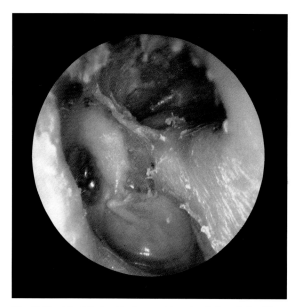

Fig. 9.18 Modified radical mastoid cavity (left ear). In this patient there is a small mastoid cavity located posteriorly in the attic area.

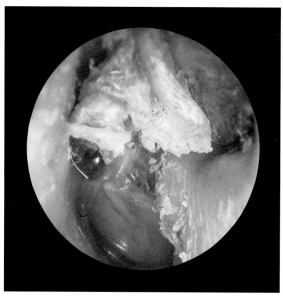

Fig. 9.19 Impacted mastoid cavity. This is the same patient as shown in Figure 9.18. Over time, the mastoid cavity has become filled with wax and desquamated keratin debris.

typical appearance of a modified radical mastoid cavity.

The posterior bony canal wall is not lowered in a simple or cortical mastoidectomy, so that the cavity is not available for inspection.

Therapeutic guidelines

The normal rate of epithelial migration of the external auditory canal may be insufficient to cleanse a large mastoid cavity of wax and epithelial debris. For this reason a mastoid cavity may require cleaning and debridement as frequently as every 6 months—more often if it is moist or infected—to remove any accumulated cerumen and keratin debris (Fig. 9.19). Generally speaking it is advisable to keep water out of a mastoid cavity, to avoid the possibility of a secondary infection.

The cleaning of a mastoid cavity should be undertaken with extreme care by someone with a thorough knowledge of the underlying anatomical structures, and ideally this procedure should be left to a specialist. The bone overlying the facial nerve may have been eroded by disease or removed during surgery, thereby rendering the facial nerve vulnerable to damage during instrumentation. The stapes footplate may be exposed and, in some cases, the bone overlying the lateral semi-circular canal may also be absent. Careless instrumentation in these two areas may render the patient extremely dizzy. It is prudent to clean mastoid cavities using a microscope which will provide both magnification and brilliant illumination.

INFECTED MASTOID CAVITY

In about 75% of cases, the cavity created following a radical or modified radical mastoid exploration becomes lined with healthy skin, causing little bother to the patient. If, however, respiratory mucosa lines the cavity, the postoperative result is a troublesome moist cavity, which is prone to infection following upper respiratory tract infections or the entry of water (Figs 9.20 and 9.21).

Symptoms

The discharge from these cavities is usually painless but foul-smelling. Pain, vertigo and a

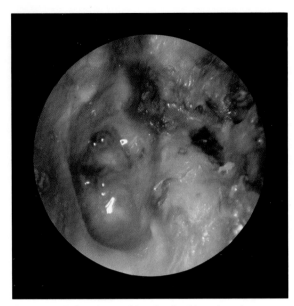

Fig. 9.20   Infected mastoid cavity. In this patient the
mastoid cavity is filled with infected wax and keratin debris.
A considerable quantity of mucopurulent discharge is present
over the tympanic membrane (left ear).

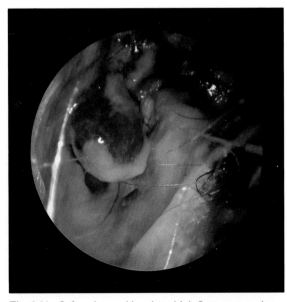

Fig. 9.21   Infected mastoid cavity with inflammatory polyp.
In this patient the infection in the mastoid cavity is caused by
an infected mass of granulation tissue, which is visible as a red
polyp (right ear).

sudden increase in hearing loss may indicate a
significant extension of infection beyond the
cavity.

Therapeutic guidelines

An infected mastoid cavity must be carefully
cleaned, either by dry-mopping using cotton
wool-tipped applicators or preferably by suction
under the operating microscope. A swab should
be taken for bacterial culture and sensitivity, as
well as fungal culture.

In this condition the pathogenic bacteria most
frequently encountered are Gram-negative
bacilli, especially *Proteus*, *Pseudomonas* species
and *Escherichia coli* species. Appropriate topical
and, in some cases, systemic antibiotics are
indicated.

In cases where the infection is persistent, the
patient should be referred for a specialist
opinion.

It should be emphasized that long-standing
chronic infection in the external or middle ear
can predispose, albeit rarely, to development of a
malignant tumour. This is one of the few areas
where there seems to be a causal relationship
between chronic infection and neoplasm.

FENESTRATION CAVITY

Until the rediscovery of stapes surgery for
otosclerosis in the 1950s, the only successful
operation to improve hearing in otosclerosis was
fenestration of the lateral semi-circular canal. In
this procedure an artificial window into the inner
ear was fashioned by thinning the bone of the
lateral semi-circular canal and covering it with a
rotation skin flap. This was combined with a
limited mastoid exploration, ensuring that there
was no obstruction to sound conduction into the
perilymph. The tympanic membrane was placed
against the upper border of the oval window
niche and acted as a barrier to prevent sound
reaching the round window.

Since a fenestrated ear closely resembles a
modified radical mastoid cavity, it is important to
obtain a sufficiently detailed history to avoid
confusion. A patient suffering from otosclerosis
will often give a family history of deafness and
have no history of preoperative ear infections. In
the fenestrated ear, the lateral semi-circular canal

is always at risk from injudicious instrumentation during wax removal and many patients become vertiginous even if great care is exercised. Patients with fenestration cavities require continuing supervision and aural toilet to prevent the accumulation of wax and epithelial debris which can predispose to secondary infection. Although this operation is no longer performed, there are still many people in the community with fenestration cavities.

POST-STAPEDECTOMY

The primary surgical treatment for otosclerosis nowadays is stapedectomy. In this operation, the conductive deafness caused by fixation of the stapes footplate in the oval window niche as a result of otosclerosis is overcome by partial or total removal of the stapes footplate. The continuity of the ossicular chain is restored either by using the patient's own stapes crura, or, more commonly, by means of an artificial prosthesis made of metal or plastic which is attached to the long process of the incus and connects with the vestibule. The oval window niche is usually sealed using a free graft of fat or vein to prevent perilymph leakage into the middle ear.

In an unusually thin tympanic membrane, the wire loop of a prosthesis may be seen. More commonly, a small amount of bone has been curetted from the posterosuperior canal wall during surgery to improve exposure. When the tympanomeatal flap is replaced, the annulus lies free. This is often the only visual clue to a previous stapedectomy (Figs 9.22–9.24).

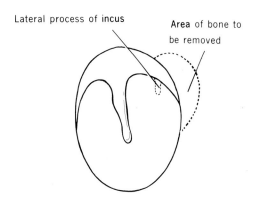
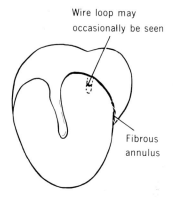

Pre operative appearance   Post operative appearance

Fig. 9.22 The area of bone usually removed to improve access to the stapes during a stapedectomy is illustrated.

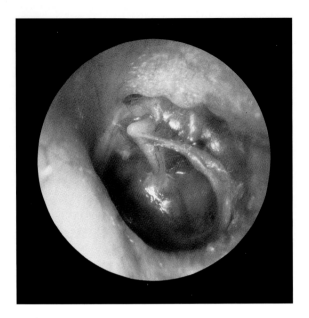

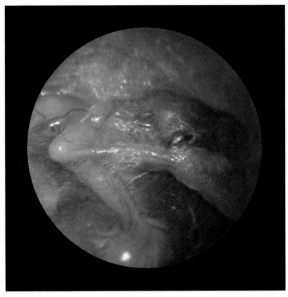

Fig. 9.24   Post-stapedectomy—higher magnification. This is the same patient as illustrated in Figure 9.23. The detail of the wire attached to the long process of the incus is more clearly seen at this higher magnification (left ear).

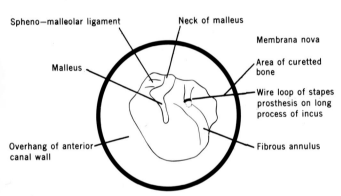

Spheno—malleolar ligament

Neck of malleus

Membrana nova

Malleus

Area of curetted bone

Wire loop of stapes prosthesis on long process of incus

Overhang of anterior canal wall

Fibrous annulus

Fig. 9.23   Post-stapedectomy (unusual appearance). In this patient an extremely large amount of bone has been removed from the posterosuperior quadrant. The small wire of the artificial stapes prosthesis crimped on the end of the long process of the incus is visible through the tympanic membrane (left ear).

10. Therapeutic principles

GENERAL CONSIDERATIONS

The successful management of any patient with a disorder of the ear demands both the ability to arrive at an accurate diagnosis and an understanding of the medical and surgical principles of treatment. The broad aim of any treatment regime is to bring rapid symptomatic relief and to institute those specific measures which will halt the disease process, thereby encouraging healing and the restoration of normal structure and function. The specific goals in managing a diseased ear are to achieve a safe, dry, symptom-free ear with good hearing and normal vestibular function.

The selection and use of drugs in the treatment of ear disease is based on established pharmacological and bacteriological principles tempered by clinical experience. Whilst some drug combinations may appear to be at variance with strict theoretical considerations, they may, nevertheless, prove useful in clinical practice. Even when there is a lack of experimental or controlled clinical data to support a particular drug regime, it may be in use simply because it is safe, effective and has stood the test of time.

The principles of treatment of infections in the ear consist, where appropriate, of debridement, drainage, the identification of the causative organism and the selection of a suitable antimicrobial given in an appropriate dosage for an adequate period of time. The initial antimicrobial of choice and the route of administration depend on the severity and location of the infective process and may be modified in the light of laboratory culture and sensitivity studies.

In many disorders of the inner ear, beyond diagnosis with the otoscope and therefore outside the scope of this text, precise pathogenesis is unclear and the treatment is therefore empirical and often based on clinical experience alone. The cause of troublesome episodic vertigo, for example, may be unclear even after exhaustive investigations, but if an inner ear disorder is suspected, symptomatic treatment with labyrinthine sedatives such as prochlorperazine (Stemetil), dimenhydrinate (Dramamine), or diazepam (Valium) or with a diuretic such as hydrochlorothiazide is frequently beneficial.

At the present time there are no proven specific medications for most causes of tinnitus or inner ear deafness. In some instances of sudden deafness, systemic vasodilators and corticosteroids may be used on the assumption that a vascular or viral disorder is responsible.

DISEASES OF THE EXTERNAL AUDITORY CANAL

Wax removal

Softening agents are of great value when hard wax completely occludes the external auditory canal. Sodium bicarbonate ear drops (sodium bicarbonate 5 g, glycerine 30 ml and purified water to 100 ml) is the most effective and efficient ceruminolytic preparation. Those ceruminolytic preparations which contain organic solvents such as turpentine are totally ineffective and should never be used as they may irritate the skin of the external canal and cause a severe contact dermatitis.

Otitis externa

Inflammatory conditions of the skin of the external auditory canal may be due to a primary bacterial, viral or fungal infection, or can result from eczema, psoriasis, seborrhoeic dermatitis and other generalized dermatological disorders.

In chronic otitis externa it is not uncommon to find more than one factor responsible and treatment of this condition can be both prolonged and difficult.

The aim of treatment in otitis externa is to make the environment within the canal less hospitable to the organism by removing secretions and debris which will act as a culture material (debridement), by altering the pH of the canal to an acidic pH in which pathogenic bacteria are incapable of surviving (using boric acid, aluminium acetate or acetic acid drops), and the use of a suitable topical antibiotic preparation.

Careful cleansing of the external canal and the reduction of meatal oedema will generally relieve discomfort; however, in severe cases, an oral analgesic may be required to abolish pain effectively. All purulent secretions and epithelial debris must be removed from the ear canal if topical antibiotic or anti-inflammatory treatment is to be effective. This can be especially difficult if the meatal skin is oedematous and the lumen virtually obliterated. Dry-mopping with a cotton wool-tipped probe and microsuction are both commonly employed.

Although water itself can precipitate otitis externa, in some patients keratin and debris can be successfully cleared by syringing, providing the tympanic membrane is intact and the ear is scrupulously dried afterwards. Whichever method of debridement is used, it cannot be over-emphasized that it is fruitless to attempt treatment with topical anti-inflammatory or antibiotic drops unless the ear canal has been thoroughly cleaned beforehand.

Hygroscopic agents such as aluminium acetate ear drops 13% or ichthymol in glycerine impregnated on a $\frac{1}{4}$ or $\frac{1}{2}$ inch (0.5 or 1 cm) ribbon gauze or Pope Otowick are useful for the reduction of the canal skin oedema and its associated discomfort.

A number of simple and compound anti-inflammatory, anti-infective preparations are available for the treatment of otitis externa. Ear drops, ointment or impregnated wicks may be selected after thorough cleansing of the external meatus. Since Gram-negative bacteria (especially *Pseudomonas aeruginosa*) are almost always cultured from swabs sent to the laboratory, the necessity of culture studies has been questioned. These studies, however, are valuable for they may reveal the presence of unsuspected bacteria or fungi resistant to the medication initially chosen.

While compound formulations containing an antimicrobial agent together with a corticosteroid may be criticized on theoretical grounds, in practice these preparations are often extremely useful in eradicating bacteria and reducing inflammatory oedema.

There is no place whatsoever for drops containing mild analgesics or local anaesthetics. These may irritate the already inflamed skin of the ear canal and, if analgesia is necessary, it should be given systemically.

Topical anti-inflammatory preparations

Topical steroids such as betamethasone sodium phosphate 0.1% (Betnesol) or triamcinolone 0.1% (Synalar) will often prevent florid otitis externa in patients with a tendency to eczematous inflammation of the canal skin. These may be given as drops or gently applied as an ointment. They are also useful in the management of neurodermatitis and itchy ear.

Topical antibacterial preparations

There are many ear drops which are useful for treating bacterial infections of the ear canal. Compound preparations containing corticosteroids or an antifungal agent are often used as initial therapy. They should not be used indefinitely, since the prolonged use of antibiotic ear drops, especially those containing neomycin, may predispose to secondary otomycosis or to the development of a sensitivity reaction to the medication itself.

In some patients topical ear drops which contain acids or alcohol may cause burning when placed in the ear. If this happens it is advisable to prescribe a similar ophthalmic preparation which has a neutral vehicle.

Some useful topical otic preparations
Chloramphenicol otic 0.5% in propylene glycol;
★ Colistin sulphate 0.3%, neomycin sulphate 0.33%, hydrocortisone acetate 1.0% (Colomycin otic);
Framycetin sulphate 0.5% (Framygen);
Gentamicin sulphate 0.3% (Genticin);
★ Gentamicin sulphate 0.3% and hydrocortisone acetate 1% (Gentisone HC);
Neomycin sulphate 0.5%, polymyxin B sulphate, hydrocortisone 1% (Cortisporin);
Neomycin sulphate 0.5%, betamethasone sodium phosphate 0.1% (Betnesol-N);
Tetracycline ointment 1% (Achromycin);
Neomycin, gramicidin, nystatin, triamcinolone in Plastibase (R) (Tri-Adcorty1 Otic);
Hydrocortisone, neomycin, polymyxin B sulphate (Otosporin);
Dexamethasone, framycetin, gramicidin ointment (Sofradex);
★ Highly recommended by the authors of this book.

Antifungal agents
Primary or secondary fungal infections of the external ear (otomycosis) are usually caused by varieties of *Candida* and *Aspergillus* species and are often difficult to treat. Chemical antifungal agents such as gentian violet and brilliant green are not always effective and colour the canal skin, potentially obscuring residual or recurrent fungal growth.

Nystatin ointment (100 000 u/g), or clotrimazole suspension 1% in propylene glycol (Canesten) are valuable topical antifungal agents for cases of *Candida* infection (clotrimazole is also highly effective against *Aspergillus*).

Amphotericin B 3% ointment (Fungilin) is useful in those cases with *Aspergillus* species.

MIDDLE EAR DISEASES

Acute otitis media
This common complication of an acute upper respiratory tract infection in children is usually treated with systemic antibiotics. The aim of treatment is to eradicate the acute bacterial infection and relieve pain while at the same time preventing the development of complications by restoring normal eustachian tube function as speedily as possible. For these reasons, a nasal decongestant and a systemic analgesic should also be administered. Because *Streptococcus pneumoniae* and *Haemophilus influenzae* are the pathogens most often responsible, amoxycillin trihydrate or cefaclor (capsules or elixir) is the initial treatment of choice. With the increasing frequency of beta-lactamase-producing bacteria, the use of the specific beta-lactamase inhibitor clavulanic acid in conjunction with amoxycillin trihydrate (Augmentin or Clavulin) is becoming increasingly more advisable. A combination of trimethoprim and sulphamethoxazole (Septrin or Bactrim) is a suitable and less expensive alternative.

Topical antibiotic treatment is ineffective if the tympanic membrane is intact, but becomes of value if a perforation occurs or in an ear which is being artificially ventilated by a grommet (tympanostomy tube).

Chronic suppurative otitis media
The initial treatment of persistent or recurrent middle ear infection begins with thorough aural toilet to remove debris and purulent exudate from the external canal so that the tympanic membrane, or what remains of it, can be inspected. This can be achieved using a cotton wool-tipped probe; however, suction under the operating microscope (microdebridement) is the preferred technique.

During microdebridement, swabs should be taken for culture and sensitivity studies. Topical antibacterial preparations containing neomycin or gentamicin can be instilled into the middle ear but prolonged treatment with ear drops must be accompanied by regular aural toilet to effect an improvement. It goes without saying that the patient should take extreme care to keep the ear dry and not allow water to enter the external canal. Steps should also be taken to investigate and, if necessary, treat any coexisting nasal obstruction or sinus disease.

The definitive treatment of the chronically

discharging ear depends on whether a cholesteatoma is present within the middle ear cleft. In patients with tubotympanic disease, in which cholesteatoma is not a feature of the pathological process, intensive local treatment, which may include aural toilet, the excision of polypoid or granular mucosa from the middle ear and therapy with appropriate topical and occasionally systemic antibiotics, will often eradicate infection and produce a healthy, dry ear.

In most cases of chronic suppurative otitis media, the organisms encountered include *Pseudomonas aeruginosa*, *Proteus*, *Staphylococcus aureus* and *Streptococcus*. For this reason, no single topical otic preparation is satisfactory for all cases. Initially, it is advisable to use a combined preparation containing a mixture of antibiotics to cover these organisms. Neomycin is effective against *Staph. aureus* and *Proteus*. Polymyxin B and polymyxin E (colistin) are generally effective against most Gram-negative organisms but not against *Proteus*, *Bacillus fragilis* or the Gram-positive organisms.

In those cases of treatment failure in which a foul smell is encountered, the possibility of an anaerobe such as *Bacteroides* should be considered. In this case, the use of chloramphenicol ear drops may be advisable.

Tympanoplastic surgery to restore hearing by reconstructing defects in the tympanic membrane or ossicular chain can be undertaken after the infection has been completely eradicated.

If a cholesteatoma is seen or suspected, and atticoantral disease is diagnosed, tympano-mastoid surgery is usually necessary to remove the cholesteatoma from the middle ear and mastoid air cells, thereby preventing the possibility of serious intracranial complications. After exenterating disease from the mastoid air cells, a cavity is created which can readily be inspected and cleaned via the external auditory canal.

Radical mastoid surgery may be required, but whenever possible steps are taken to preserve or restore elements of the tympanic membrane and the ossicular chain to produce the best possible hearing result. Nevertheless, it is always safer for the patient to accept a healthy cavity with some hearing rather than run the risk of developing further disease behind an intact posterior canal wall and an apparently normal tympanic membrane. A suitable hearing aid will help those patients who are left with a conductive hearing loss following mastoid surgery

THE EUSTACHIAN TUBE

The health of the middle ear cleft is intimately dependent on a normally functioning eustachian tube. Since the majority of upper respiratory tract infections are primarily viral in origin, the routine use of systemic antibiotics will not prevent tubal occlusion or ascending infection. Eustachian dysfunction can also result from nasal allergy or vasomotor instability and systemic or topical drugs may be an appropriate adjunct to the treatment of some ear disorders.

Topical nasal decongestants

Saline sniffs (sodium chloride 0.9%) are simple and often effective in clearing the nose of mucus. Topical sympathomimetics reduce the thickness of the nasal mucosa by vasoconstriction but prolonged usage can cause rebound obstruction or even permanent damage to the nasal cilia, leading to atrophic rhinitis medicamentosa.

Ephedrine nose drops 0.5% in glucose–saline are safe, for they do not interfere with ciliary action. However, these drops may be difficult to obtain commercially.

Xylometazoline (Otrivine) and oxymetazoline (Afrazine, Iliadin) are more potent and longer-acting, but may, with prolonged use, result in the development of rebound nasal obstruction (rhinitis medicamentosa).

Oral nasal decongestants

These may be of value in the treatment of secretory otitis media (glue ear) in children or adults. Most are a combination of an anti-histamine with a sympathomimetic and are therefore capable of causing drowsiness.

Examples include brompheniramine maleate with phenylephrine hydrochloride and phenyl-propanolamine hydrochloride (Dimetapp) and pseudoephedrine with triprolidine (Actifed).

OTOTOXICITY

A considerable variety of drugs can cause auditory and vestibular damage. The aminoglycosides, widely used systemically for the treatment of severe Gram-negative sepsis and topically in the management of severe burns, have a tendency to be ototoxic, especially if renal function is impaired. Although in experimental animals the introduction of aminoglycosides into the middle ear is associated with inner ear damage, it is fortunate that topical aminoglycoside ear drops in man have not been associated with ototoxicity.

11. Hearing tests

A pure tone sound can be objectively quantified by its intensity, which is measured in decibels (dB), and by its frequency, which is measured in hertz (cycles per second). These two objective parameters are perceived subjectively as loudness and pitch respectively. The normal human ear is able to perceive sound over a fairly wide range of frequencies from 32 to 16 000 hertz (Hz). This range extends over nine octaves; from three octaves below middle C to six octaves above.

In the middle frequencies, (500–4000 Hz) the human ear is capable of accommodating in comfort a wide range of intensities up to 100 dB. In visual terms, less energy is required to provide an audible sound than is generated by a candle which can be seen on a dark night at a distance of 200 metres, and yet the ear can withstand sounds which have the equivalent visual intensity of bright sunlight. Because of this huge range, intensity is measured on a logarithmic scale and quantified as decibels (one tenth of a Bel). Ten decibels is 10 times as loud as zero decibels, and twenty decibels is 100 times as intense as zero decibels.

Hearing, or an individual's ability to hear sound, is measured by means of an audiometer. This is a device which produces pure tone sounds of known frequency, which can be changed at the tester's will (usually in half octave steps), and known intensity, which can also be adjusted by the tester (usually in 5 dB increments). The act of testing hearing is termed audiometry, and the results of the hearing test are plotted on a form called an audiogram.

PURE TONE THRESHOLD AUDIOMETRY

An individual's ability to hear sound conducted by air (*air conduction*) is tested by presenting sounds to the ear via an earphone. Air conduction testing assesses the entire auditory system (i.e. the transmission of sound down the ear canal, through the tympanic membrane, middle and inner ears).

Bone conduction testing bypasses the ear canal and the middle ear by directly vibrating the mastoid process with a bone oscillator (vibrator). These vibrations are then carried through the bones of the skull to the inner ear where they stimulate the cochlea. Bone conduction tests are used to measure the thresholds of hearing of the inner ear.

The most common type of audiometry performed is pure tone threshold audiometry, which measures the level of intensity at which the patient can just perceive sound. The threshold of hearing is the intensity (in decibels) for a given frequency at which the tone is heard in 50% of presentations.

Pure tone audiometric testing usually starts with an assessment of the responses to air conduction (using headphones) at 1000 Hz in the better ear. The test begins by instructing the subject to respond to the faintest sound that they can hear. The intensity is set on the audiometer to a level at which the sound can be easily heard, and the tone is presented. If the sound is heard, then the intensity is reduced by 10 dB. If the sound is again heard, the intensity is reduced by a further 10 dB, and so on until the sound is no longer heard.

When the subject fails to respond, the intensity is increased by 5 dB until the sound is again heard, and once again, the intensity is dropped by 10 dB until it is no longer heard. Because 5 dB is quite a large change in intensity, the subject is usually quite clear whether or not they hear the sound.

The intensity level at which the patient hears the sound in 50% of presentations is recorded on the audiogram in decibels of hearing level (dBHL) as the 'threshold' for 1000 Hz. This testing procedure is then repeated and the results plotted on the audiogram at 2000, 4000, 6000 and 8000 Hz and then at 250 and 500 Hz in order to determine the thresholds of hearing for these frequencies.

Because all of the speech sounds (both consonants and vowels) used for normal communication occur within the frequency range from 250 to 8000 Hz, the frequencies outside of this range are not routinely tested. The testing procedure is then repeated on the other ear to complete the air conduction audiogram.

The testing procedure may then be repeated using a bone conduction oscillator at the frequencies 250, 500, 1000, 2000 and 4000 Hz to measure the bone conduction thresholds.

The audiogram

The results of pure tone threshold audiometry are usually plotted on an audiogram form. Figure 11.1 shows a normal audiogram. On an audiogram, the frequency of sound (in Hz) is

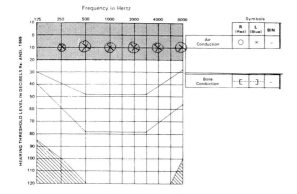

Fig. 11.1 A normal pure tone air conduction audiogram. The circles show the test results for the right ear and the Xs the results for the left ear (note the key to the codes).

displayed across the top of the form in octave bands from 250 Hz (the lowest frequency tested) on the left, to 8000 Hz (the highest frequency sounds) on the right.

Audiometers are calibrated for 0 degrees hearing loss (the threshold of hearing for normal young adults) at each frequency. The intensity of the sound which the subject was just able to hear (the threshold) is represented along the vertical axis of the audiogram in decibels with the 0 dB (a very faint sound) at the top of the vertical axis and 110 dB (loud sound) at the bottom. It is customary to plot the results for the right ear using circles and the left ear using Xs. Because the symbols used to represent the various tests performed on each ear may vary from clinic to clinic, each audiogram form should include a key explaining the symbols used (Fig. 11.1).

Like most biological functions, 'normal' hearing encompasses a range which extends from −10 dB (very acute hearing) to +10 dB (less acute but still normal hearing). A hearing loss (pure tone threshold) of 15 dB or greater is considered abnormal. The severity of an individual's hearing loss can be categorized by averaging the pure tone air conduction thresholds obtained at 500, 1000 and 2000 Hz (Table 11.1)

SPEECH AUDIOMETRY

The threshold of hearing may also be assessed by performing a test known as the speech reception threshold (SRT) test which measures the lowest level at which speech is understood. In this test, bisyllabic words called spondees in which both syllables are of equal intensity (e.g. cowboy, airplane, baseball etc) are presented through the headphone in groups of four words at a given intensity. The intensity at which the next group of spondees is presented is dropped by 5 dB if the previous group was correctly identified. This procedure is continued until the intensity level at which 50% of the words are correctly heard is identified. This level is known as the speech reception threshold.

The speech reception threshold should be within 10 dB of the average pure tone threshold for the frequencies of 500, 1000, and 2000 Hz. The SRT is primarily used to confirm the results of pure tone threshold testing. Higher SRT levels (levels greater than 10 dB of the average pure tone threshold for the frequencies of 500, 1000, and 2000 Hz) may occur in patients who have problems with speech discrimination (reduced clarity of spoken sounds). In contrast, the SRT in patients with functional hearing loss (malingerers) may be better than the level which would be expected based on their pure tone audiogram.

SPEECH DISCRIMINATION

The tests described previously are tests which only measure the thresholds of hearing, i.e. the quietest sounds that can be heard. Normal listening is done at levels comfortably louder than these thresholds, and in addition, normal listening depends upon another important characteristic of hearing, known as discrimination; this is the ability to distinguish correctly one sound from another. Discrimination is tested audiometrically by means of the speech discrimination test which measures the amount of difficulty in understanding speech presented under favourable listening conditions.

In the speech discrimination test, monosyllabic words with similar sounds are presented at the patient's most comfortable listening level (MCL) (usually 35–40 dB above the speech reception threshold) and the subject is asked to repeat the words back. Words like cat, hat, bat, sat and thin, fin and bin are used in this test. These words are presented in specially constructed word lists which are equivalent in difficulty to each other. Usually 25 words are presented and the score is expressed as a percentage of the words correctly repeated. A normal score in a quiet background is 91% or more correct.

An abnormality in this speech discrimination test suggests that there is a problem within either the nerve of hearing or that part of the brain which deals with hearing. In a purely conductive hearing loss, the speech discrimination scores are usually normal as there is no pathology in the neural pathways with this type of loss. Table 11.2 presents a general guideline to the amount of difficulty in understanding normal conversation that patients with different speech discrimination

scores will experience.

AUDIOGRAM INTERPRETATION

The extent and cause of a hearing loss can usually be determined from an examination of the audiogram. The severity of the hearing loss can be determined by averaging the pure tone air conduction thresholds obtained at 500, 1000 and 2000 Hz (Table 11.1).

The amount of difficulty that an individual is likely to experience in understanding conversation can be determined by the speech discrimination score (Table 11.2).

If the hearing loss is purely sensorineural (i.e. no abnormality in the middle ear sound conducting mechanism), then the air conduction and bone conduction thresholds will be the same (Fig. 11.2). The two most common types of sensorineural hearing loss can be diagnosed from

Table 11.1 A simple method for classifying the severity of hearing loss

Average threshold level (dB) (at 500, 1000 and 2000 Hz)	Severity of the hearing loss
−10–15	normal
16–25	slight
26–40	mild
41–55	moderate
56–70	moderately severe
71–90	severe
91+	profound

From Katz J 1985 Handbook of Clinical Audiology, Williams & Wilkins, New York.

Table 11.2 The amount of difficulty in understanding normal conversation based on the measured speech discrimination score

Percentage score	Level of difficulty in understanding speech
91–100	normal
76–90	slight difficulty
61–75	moderate difficulty
51–60	poor
0–50	very poor

From Katz J 1985 Handbook of Clinical Audiology, Williams & Wilkins, New York.

the shape of the audiogram. In presbyacusis (a slowly progressive, initially high frequency sensorineural hearing loss, that results from ageing changes within the inner ear) the lower frequencies are usually normal and the audiogram slopes downward in the higher frequencies (Fig. 11.3). In patients with a noise induced sensorineural hearing loss (industrial or occupational deafness) the hearing loss is maximal at 4000 Hz (Fig. 11.4).

In a conductive hearing loss, the air conduction thresholds will be below the bone conduction thresholds (an air bone gap) (Fig. 11.4).

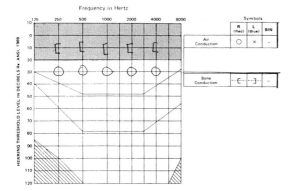

Fig. 11.2 A pure tone air and bone conduction audiogram showing a conductive hearing loss in the right ear. Note the normal bone conduction thresholds (the open brackets) and the decreased air conduction thresholds (the circles). The difference between the bone and air conduction thresholds is called an air–bone gap, and is indicative of a conductive hearing loss.

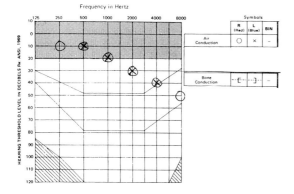

Fig. 11.3 Presbyacusis. A pure tone audiogram showing the typical high frequency sensorineural hearing loss that develops in some patients with ageing. The low frequencies are normal with a sloping (gradually increasing) hearing loss in the higher frequencies.

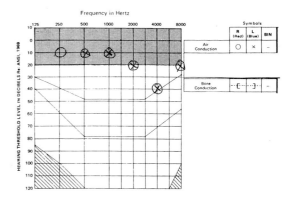

Fig. 11.4 Noise induced sensorineural hearing loss. This audiogram shows the typical appearance of noise induced sensorineural hearing loss. Note the high frequency hearing loss which is maximal at 4000 Hz (the 4000 Hz dip).

MIDDLE EAR FUNCTION TESTING

If a conductive hearing loss is suspected or found, it is valuable to know whether this is due to fluid in the middle ear, or if there is a problem with the ossicular chain. The clinical appearance of the tympanic membrane does not always give a clue to the cause of the conductive hearing loss. The technique of tympanometry is used to unravel this situation.

Tympanometry is based on the observation that if a sound is introduced into a sealed external auditory canal, some of the sound will be absorbed by the middle ear, and some will remain in the external canal. If the same plug which is sealing off the external ear canal contains, in addition to the sound source and the probe microphone which measures the amount of sound remaining in the ear canal, a tube leading to a pressure pump which allows the air pressure within the external canal to be raised or lowered, then the ability of the middle ear to absorb sound can be measured at differing air pressure (usually over a range from +400 to −400 mm of water).

It is well know that the sensitivity of the ear to sound is dependent on the pressure of the air within the middle ear relative to the pressure of the surrounding atmosphere. Clearing the ears when either ascending or descending in an aeroplane makes sounds much louder.

Tympanometry measures two parameters, the mobility of the tympanic membrane (compliance) and the pressure within the middle ear. In automatic tympanometry, the sound pressure level in the external ear canal is plotted over continuous changes in the air pressure within the external canal. The equipment required for this type of automatic tympanometry is relatively simple and highly automated. A probe with a rubber tip is inserted into the ear canal, and once an airtight seal of the canal is obtained, the device automatically changes the air pressure within the canal and prints out the results.

In a normal ear, the sound absorption (i.e. the compliance of the middle ear) is greatest at, or close to, atmospheric pressure, with a sharp fall off within 50 mm of water on either side (Fig. 11.5). The top of the peak (i.e. the point at which the tympanic membrane is most responsive to sound and at which the hearing is most sensitive) occurs when the air pressure in the ear canal (i.e. atmospheric pressure) and in the middle ear are at the same level.

If there is a significant negative pressure within the middle ear, the peak will be shifted to the left (the negative pressure side of the chart) (Fig. 11.6). If the middle ear is filled with fluid, (as happens in serous and mucoid otitis media) there is no peak and the tracing is flat (Fig. 11.7).

Tympanometry does not require any responses from the patient, and consequently this technique is a useful way of measuring middle ear function in patients who are either difficult to test or unresponsive.

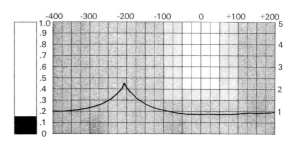

Fig. 11.6 A tympanogram showing negative pressure in the middle ear. When there is negative pressure within the middle ear, the peak is shifted to the left (the negative pressure side of the chart).

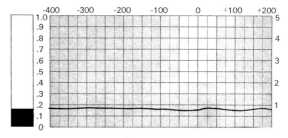

Fig. 11.7 A tympanogram showing fluid in the middle ear. When the middle ear is filled with fluid, (as happens in serous and mucoid otitis media) there is no peak and the tracing is flat.

AURAL REHABILITATION

Hearing loss can be one of the most insidious and debilitating handicaps. Many hearing impaired adults will deny that they have any problem with their hearing, blaming instead those who speak to them for mumbling or speaking softly. These individuals may become withdrawn and isolated from their friends and family. The first step in breaking this chain of events is the establishment in the patient's mind of the fact that a hearing loss is really present.

While the overwhelming majority of people with hearing impairment are still able to use their sense of hearing for communication, there remain a large number of adults (and some children) who have a hearing loss of such a significant degree that some form of assistance to hearing (termed aural rehabilitation) is required for them to function fully in everyday life.

Aural rehabilitation can take three major directions: another sense can be substituted for the sense of sound, all sounds can be amplified,

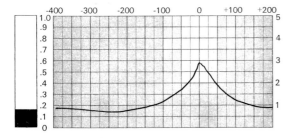

Fig. 11.5 A normal tympanogram. In a normal ear, the sound absorption (i.e. the compliance of the middle ear) is greatest at, or close to, atmospheric pressure, with a sharp fall off within 50 mm of water on either side. Note the top of the peak (i.e. the point at which the tympanic membrane is most responsive to sound and at which the hearing is most sensitive) occurs when the air pressure in the ear canal (i.e. atmospheric pressure) and in the middle ear are at the same level.

or a specific sound of interest can be amplified. A flashing light can be substituted for a doorbell, a hearing aid can be provided to amplify all sounds, or an amplifier can be provided for a telephone headset. Each of these have their role, although for the majority of the hearing impaired, the amplification of sound, either general or specific is the preferred choice, with a sensory substitution being reserved for special instances, particularly for the severely hard of hearing.

The hearing aid

The hearing aid consists of a microphone, an amplifier and a miniature loudspeaker (commonly called a receiver). It can be likened to a highly miniaturized public address system. Today, most hearing aids are worn at ear level, either in the ear (an ITE aid) or behind the ear (a BTE aid).

The ITE hearing aid is the most commonly prescribed device at the present time and consists of a fairly large ear mould which sits in the conchal bowl and extends into the outer part of the ear canal. The mould of an ITE aid is large enough to contain a battery to power the device, a microphone to pick up sounds, an amplifier and a speaker (receiver). ITE hearing aids are relatively inconspicuous and have the advantage that sounds come to the microphone fairly naturally, collected by the pinna which protects it somewhat from unwanted sounds behind the head.

The BTE hearing aid has the microphone and associated electronics in a slim curved container which hangs by a hook over the ear, with a tube leading to an ear mould, which pipes the sound into the ear canal. It is possible to fit more electronics into a BTE aid, and therefore produce a more sophisticated electronic device. The BTE hearing aid is in fact usually quite inconspicuous, particularly in long haired individuals, because the mould is much smaller than that of an ITE hearing aid, and the ear mould is often the only visible part of the device.

The most powerful hearing aids are the body aids. This type of hearing aid is usually reserved for the severely hard of hearing due to the body aid's less aesthetic appearance.

Hearing aids can to some extent be adjusted to match the characteristics of the hearing loss. Nevertheless, most hearing aids emphasize the high frequency sounds more than the low frequency sounds because the consonants (those sounds which distinguish the words of everyday listening) are high pitched, whereas the vowels which are lower in pitch are also relatively loud.

One of the basic problems with hearing aids is that they make all sounds louder and not just the sound which the listener is interested in, i.e. they amplify background noise as well as speech. People with sensorineural hearing loss already have difficulty in blocking out unwanted sounds, and for these reasons, hearing aids are most helpful in relatively quiet surroundings.

Assistive devices for the hearing impaired

Many communicative situations are filled with distractions that can seriously interfere with the listening process, even for individuals who have normal hearing. The effects of unwanted background noise, distance from the source of the sound, poor room acoustics, and reverberation can create an insurmountable obstacle for the hearing impaired. In response to these problems, a series of electronic devices have been developed which can improve the ability of the hearing impaired person to communicate in specific listening situations.

Assistive devices are classified into several categories including: assistive listening devices (e.g. personal amplifiers), assistive alerting devices (e.g. loud bells or buzzers to alert the listener to sounds around them), assistive signalling devices (e.g. flashing lights or vibrating devices to signal an event or an emergency), telecommunications devices (e.g. facsimile machines and computers with modems) and informing devices (e.g. closed captioning for television).

Appendix 1

SPEECH AND HEARING CHECKLIST

This checklist is reprinted from the brochure *Speech and Hearing Checklist for the Family Physician* by kind permission of the Ontario Speech and Hearing Association. The preparation and publication of *Speech and Hearing Checklist for the Family Physician* was sponsored by the Harmonize for Speech Fund of the Ontario District Association of Chapters of the Society for the Preservation and Encouragement of Barber-shop Quartet Singing in America Inc.

Introduction

The first 5 years of a child's life are critical in the development of speech and hearing. The child who enters school with a communication disorder has a much greater chance of experiencing failure which can permeate through the entire school career. The early detection of speech and hearing problems can minimize these problems by allowing early intervention. If the answer to any of the age-appropriate questions on this checklist is *no* then referral for a speech and language assessment is indicated.

Birth to 6 months

Does the child:

1. Startle to loud sudden noises?
2. Sometimes stir or awaken when sleeping quietly and someone makes a loud noise?
3. Does the 3- to 6-month-old child stop moving when called?

6 to 12 months

Does the child:

1. Turn towards a sound when his/her name is called?
2. Babble, laugh or make sounds like 'ga-ga', 'ma-ma' or 'ba-ba'?

12 to 15 months

Does the child:

1. Repeat sounds?
2. Understand some simple phrases like 'come here', 'don't touch'?
3. Recognize the telephone or the doorbell ringing etc.?

15 to 18 months

Can the child:

1. Say 4–6 different words?
2. Tell you what he/she wants by pointing and saying a word?
3. Understand phrases like 'give me that' when gestures are used?
4. Recognize the names of common objects like 'ball', 'table', 'bed', 'car'?
5. Use the names of familiar things like 'water', 'cup', 'biscuit', 'clock'?

18 to 24 months

Can the child:

1. Use 2-word combinations?
2. Say about 20 or more words?
3. Use words to express physical needs?
4. Follow simple directions like 'sit down', 'give me the ball'?
5. Point to an appropriate picture when you say 'show me the dog (hat, man, etc.)'?

2 to 3 years

Can the child:

1. Use 3-word sentences?
2. Tell a story or express his/her feelings in words?
3. Remember some recently past events?
4. Count to 3?
5. Tell you his/her first and last name?
6. Can people outside the family understand 40–50% of what he/she says?

3 to 4 years

Does the child:

1. Use 4–5-word sentences?
2. Tell a story?
3. Ask a lot of questions?
4. Repeat a sentence of 8–9 syllables: 'We are going to buy some sweets'.
5. Name 3 colours?
6. Use plurals like 'toys', 'balls'?
7. Repeat 3 or 4 numbers?

4 to 5 years

1. Can he/she define 4 or more common words or tell how the objects are used (e.g. hat, dish, apples)?
2. Can he/she name a penny, 5p and 10p?
3. Do people outside the family understand 80–90% of what he/she says?
4. Does he/she like to look at books and have someone read to him/her?
5. Does he/she use I, me, you, he/she and him/her properly?

Appendix 2

TYMPANIC MEMBRANE PHOTOGRAPHY

The majority of the photographs of the external ear canal and tympanic membrane in this book were taken using a commercially available Karl Storz Hopkins Rod Tele-otoscope. The Hopkins Rod lens system was invented by Professor H. H. Hopkins, an optical engineer at the University of Reading, UK. This unique optical system utilizes special quartz rods with concave polished ends separated by small 'air lenses'. The Hopkins Rod lens system provides more efficient light transmission and increased magnification with a resulting brighter and more easily viewed image. In addition, the optical qualities of this system provide an improved resolution and a wider field of view, as well as a greater depth of field than can be obtained with conventional telescopes.

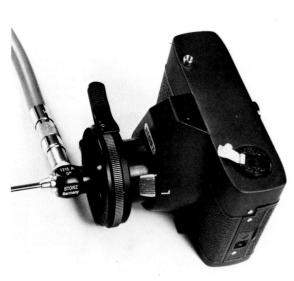

Fig. A1 The Hopkins Rod Tele-otoscope attached to the Endocamera.

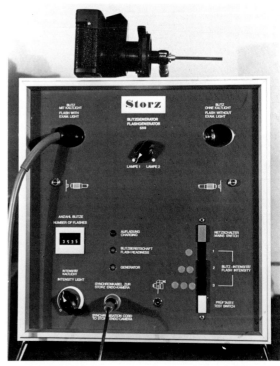

Fig. A2 The Karl Storz Tele-otoscope, Endocamera and flash generator.

The system used for the photographs in this book included a Karl Storz 4 mm outside diameter forward-viewing Hopkins Rod Tele-otoscope (model no. 1215A), and a Karl Storz (model no. 580) Endocamera (Fig. A1) which is attached to the tele-otoscope by an integral quick-connect clamp and contains a 90 mm zoom lens which is left in the L (long distance) position.

An integral electronic flash and cold light fountain (Karl Storz model no. 599C) is attached to the tele-otoscope by a fibreoptic cable (model no. 495S-SW) (Fig. A2).

Kodachrome ASA 64, daylight colour balance film (KR 135–20P) was used and photographs were taken at the no. 1 and no. 2 flash power settings.

Complete details of the technique used can be found in Hawke M 1982 Telescopic otoscopy and photography of the tympanic membrane. Journal of Otolaryngology 11: 35–39.

Appendix 3

A list of instruments recommended by the authors for use in examination of the ear. (To assist in identification, KARL STORZ Catalogue article numbers have been included.)

For illumination

Headmirror	Karl Storz	J1 076090
Gooseneck lamp with 100 Watt light bulb		
Headlight	Karl Storz	J3 087200

Probes and curettes

Jobson Horne probe 18 cm	Karl Storz	E12 152400
Wagener ear hook, extra small	Karl Storz	E12 152301
Wagener ear hook, ball end	Karl Storz	E12 152202
Buck blunt ear curette, size 1	Karl Storz	E13 153301
Buck blunt ear curette, size 2	Karl Storz	E13 153302

Suction tubes

Zoellner suction tube	Karl Storz	E21 204700
Ferguson suction tube	Karl Storz	E21 204808
Barnes suction tube	Karl Storz	203617
Spare detachable fine ends for the Zoellner and Ferguson suction tubes	Karl Storz	E21 204705
House cut-out adapter		

Forceps

Hartmann crocodile action forceps	Karl Storz	E14 161000
Hartmann ear dressing forceps	Karl Storz	E14 158500
Troeltsh ear dressing forceps	Karl Storz	E14 157000
Lucae bayonet-shaped dressing forceps	Karl Storz	E14 156000

Additional ENT examination instruments

Hartmann tongue depressor—adult	Karl Storz	MT1 740700
Hartmann tongue depressor—child	Karl Storz	MT1 740800
Thudichum nasal speculum	Karl Storz	N1 410202
Hartmann nasal speculum	Karl Storz	N1 400500

Laryngeal mirrors	Karl Storz	La Inst 1
Size 00 (8 mm)		769920
Size 2 (14 mm)		769902
Size 5 (20 mm)		769905
Spirit lamp for warming mirrors	Karl Storz	HS 815500
Hartmann ear specula	Karl Storz	E8 122004
		−122007
Bruenings modification of Siegle pneumatic speculum with 4 specula and rubber bulb	Karl Storz	E1 120400
Reiner ear syringe	Karl Storz	E9 133810

Equipment for simple clinical tests of hearing

Tuning fork with base (512 Hertz)	Karl Storz	E8 125501
Barany-Frenzel noise apparatus	Karl Storz	E9 130200

Bibliography

Basic sciences

Anson B J, Donaldson J A 1981 Surgical anatomy of the temporal bone and ear, 3rd edn. W B Saunders, Philadelphia

A complete account of temporal bone morphology, the developmental anatomy of the ear and the topography of the adult ear. Profusely illustrated with line drawings, reconstructions, dissections and photomicrographs of temporal bone sections.

Beagley H A 1981 Audiology and audiological medicine. Oxford University Press, Oxford

An excellent text of basic and applied audiology.

Friedmann I 1974 Pathology of the ear. Blackwell Scientific Publications, Oxford

A well written and readable study of the pathology of ear disease.

Hinchcliffe R, Harrison D F N (eds) 1976 Scientific foundations of otolaryngology. Wm Heinemann, London

Sections V and VI deal with the structure and function of the ear and constitute a useful introduction to scientific literature. Subjects covered include the mechanics of the auditory apparatus, eustachian tube function, impedance, the labyrinthine fluids, psychoacoustics, vestibular physiology and neurotology.

Katz J 1978 The handbook of clinical audiology, 2nd Edn. Williams & Wilkins, Baltimore, Maryland

This is one of the standard texts on audiology.

Schuknecht H F 1974 pathology of the ear. Commonwealth Fund Publications, Harvard, Massachusetts

A comprehensive description, accompanied by photomicrographs, of disease processes as they affect the ear. A useful bibliography of key papers accompanies each section.

The practice of otology

J B Booth (ed) 1987 Scott Brown's otolaryngology. Vol 3. Otology. Butterworth, London

Ballantyne J, Martin J.A.M., 1984 Deafness, 4th edn. Churchill Livingstone, Edinburgh

A useful introduction to problems of hearing disorders and an excellent and comprehensive introductory text on otology.

Ludman H 1988 Mawson's Diseases of the ear, 5th edn. Arnold, London

This is the 5th edition of one of the classic textbooks of otology.

Paparella M M, Shumrick D H (eds) 1980 Otolaryngology, 2nd Edn. Vol 2. The ear

Each volume presents a detailed account of the current practice of otology and describes current views on the diagnosis and treatment of ear discorders.

Shambaugh, G E, Glasscock, M E 1980 Surgery of the ear, 3rd edn. W B Saunders, Philadelphia

This is the third edition of one of the standard texts on surgical tretment of ear disorders.

Further reading

Senturia B H 1980 Diseases of the external ear, 2nd edn. Grune & Stratton, New York

A practical guide to the management of disorders of the external ear.

Sade J 1979 Secretory otitis media and its sequelae. Churchill Livingstone, Edinburgh

A presentation of the relevant research on secretory otitis media and its relationship to chronic otitis.

Smith G D L 1980 Chronic ear disease. Churchill Livingstone, Edinburgh

A personal view of the surgical treatment of chronic middle ear disease.

Index